Philosophy and Medicine

Revised edition

E. K. LEDERMANN, M.D., FRCPsych.

Gower

Published by
Gower Publishing Company Limited
Gower House
Croft Road
Aldershot
Hants GU11 3HR
England

Gower Publishing Company
Old Post Road
Brookfield
Vermont 05036
USA

First edition published in Great Britain in 1970 by Tavistock Publications Limited.

British Library Cataloguing in Publication Data

Ledermann, E.K.
    Philosophy and medicine. — Rev ed.
    1. Medicine — Philosophy
    I. Title
    610'.1   R723

Library of Congress Cataloging-in-Publication Data

Ledermann, E. K. (Erich Kurt), 1908-
    Philosophy and medicine.

    Includes bibliographies and index.
    1. Holistic medicine. 2. Medicine — Philosophy.
    3. Medicine and psychology. 4. Kant, Immanuel,
    1724-1804. I. Title. [DNLM: 1. Philosophy, Medical.
    W 61 L473p]
    R733.L43 1986   610'.1   86-14841

ISBN 0-566-05062-5

Printed in Great Britain at the
University Press, Cambridge

To
My Wife

Contents

FOREWORD BY DR DAVID LAMB   *page* ix

PREFACE TO THE REVISED EDITION   xi

ACKNOWLEDGEMENTS   xv

INTRODUCTION   xix

Chapter 1

Two Philosophies of Medicine

Part I   THE PHILOSOPHY OF MECHANISTIC MATERIALISM   3
    Monistic Physico-chemical Materialism   3
      The Model in Physico-chemical Materialism   7
    Monistic Biological-mechanistic Materialism   10

Part II THE PHILOSOPHY OF HOLISM   16
    Holism in Physics and Biology   17
    Holism in Medical Psychology   22
    The Holistic Principle   24
    The Holistic Principle in Medical Practice   25
      (a) Bodily Illness   25
      (b) Mental (emotional) Illness   28
    The Holistic Principle and the Material Substrate 34

Chapter II

Medicine and the 'Copernican Revolution' in Thought

Part I   KANTIAN EPISTEMOLOGY AND SCIENCE   43
    The 'Copernican Revolution' in Thought   43
    Science and Metaphysics   46
    The Relation of Body and Mind   49
    Concepts and Physical Reality   53
    The Relationship of Mechanistic Materialism and Holism
      and the Significance of the Two Principles in Biology 56
    Teleology in Young's Conception of the Brain   59

CONTENTS

Part II   KANTIAN EPISTEMOLOGY AND PSYCHOLOGICAL
        MEDICINE   62
        Theory of Psychological Medicine   62
        The Idea of a Comprehensive Behavioural Science   63
        The Idea of a Social Psychiatry   65
        The Idea of the Individual Psyche in Medical
          Psychologies   75
        Epistemological Conclusions regarding Individual Medical
          Psychology   92
        Psychic Determinism and Freedom   94
        The Evaluation of Human Relations in Medical
          Psychology   99
        Conclusion   102

Part III   KANTIAN EPISTEMOLOGY AND THE UNIFICA-
        TION OF SCIENTIFIC THOUGHT   109

Chapter III

Medicine and Ethics

Introduction   119
Medicine and Naturalistic Ethics — The Patient as Object   120
    Deterministic Psychologies   122
Medicine and Existential Ethics — The Patient as Subject   128
    The Integration of the Existential and Phenomenological
        Principles within a Medical Framework   130
    An Existential Re-Interpretation of some Central Insights
        of Medical Psychologies   142
    The Patient's Struggle for Faith   145
    The Ontologies of Sartre and Heidegger   146
    The Experience of the Body   161
Medicine based on Existential Ethics   162

AUTHOR INDEX   171

SUBJECT INDEX   173

Foreword

The biomedical revolution of the past two decades has raised fundamental questions concerning the conceptual foundations of medicine. On both sides of the Atlantic moral philosophers have become involved in some of the ethical problems which are related to the employment of scientific methods in contemporary medicine. It is also significant that Governments feel that it is proper that the moral problems arising in scientific medicine should be investigated by committees headed by philosophers. As medicine advances into new areas greater conceptual uncertainty is evident. Quite clearly both the physician and the philosopher have much to offer each other.

Yet so far philosophers have confined their attention to the ethical aspects of scientific medicine. What is now required is more discussion of the metaphysical and epistemological aspects of medicine. Perhaps one reason for the scarcity of material in this area is that few philosophers and physicians have sufficient expertise in both disciplines. It is for this reason that Dr Ledermann's book — first published in 1970 — can be hailed as an important landmark in the conceptualisation of medicine. Viewing medicine from a philosophical point of view Dr Ledermann reveals his competence in medicine and recent philosophy. The early sections of the book provide a scholarly critique of the two major philosophical approaches to medicine; mechanism and holism. These standpoints are evaluated in their own right and in terms of the forms of treatment deemed appropriate within each approach. Dr Ledermann also recognises that the theory of knowledge also lies at the heart of medical research and treatment, and that the differences between underlying philosophical standpoints actually lead to different forms of treatment. Thus the epistemological standpoint of naive realism (often associated with positivistic models of scientific practice) is contrasted with an epistemology which Ledermann derives from a Kantian theory of knowledge, and the practical implications for medical practice are likewise contrasted.

Throughout the book Dr Ledermann writes authoritatively on both medical and philosophical matters, demonstrating how the interaction between the two subjects requires constant investigation. In a very important sense *Philosophy and Medicine* is even more relevant today than it was a decade ago. The pace of scientific research in medicine has dramatically accelerated bringing with it a pressing need for an elaboration of its philosophical foundations. Moreover, in an era of competing concepts of therapy and radical departures from orthodox treatment, it is important to show exactly how philosophical beliefs influence diagnosis and prognosis. And once it is demonstrated how inferior therapy follows from bad philosophy the requirement for a rigorous examination of medicine's philosophical base is a matter of considerable urgency.

Dr David Lamb, Series Editor,
Department of Philosophy
University of Manchester
September 1986

Preface to Revised Edition

Since this book was published in 1970 its subject matter has become more and more topical. The two philosophies of medicine, mechanistic materialism and holism, appear to be in conflict: the former is taught and practiced by the established school, the latter by those who either claim to represent an alternative school or to provide a necessary complementary approach. Leading medical journals in Great Britain and in the United States of America have denied that these claims are justified.

The conflict must be resolved. The mechanists cannot eliminate the influence of the holists, as more and more people seek treatments from holistic practitioners, naturopaths, acupuncturists and others. The holists cannot replace the powerful body of medical scientific research and its applications.

This book offers a way out of this impasse. It characterizes mechanistic materialism and holism as two ways of gaining knowledge of the phenomena with which doctors are concerned. 'The philosophies of mechanistic materialism and holism are theories about the nature of the universe and its features... [They] lead to an interpretation of the patient in terms of individual parts and cause-effect relations, and in terms of wholes and holistic forces respectively.' (page 43). They are tools for gaining knowledge, provided by our cognitive minds. This clarification of medicine follows from an application of Kant's theory of knowledge.

The enquiry into the significance of the holistic principle shows that it is not only evident in those forms of treatment which call themselves 'holistic', but that it plays a vital part also in the theory and practice of the dominant school.

Although the method of scientific medicine is analytical and specific, no part of the body can be understood except by relating it to the whole of which it is a part. This relationship is teleological, the question is always what purpose a part plays for the maintenance of the whole. For instance, the function of the heart is explained as the organ which serves the purpose of supplying the organs of the body with blood, the function of the kidneys as the organ which eliminates certain waste products in the urine, and if any of these functions are disturbed, life is in danger and medical or surgical methods are employed in order to rectify the balance on which health depends. The nature of the two philosophical principles is elucidated in the following way: with the aid of mechanistic materialism medical scientific knowledge is *constituted*. The holistic principle finds expression in the scientist's *reflection* on the objects of his study. They themselves have no purpose, but, as Kant has pointed out, the scientist looks upon them *as if* they had a purpose, he uses the teleological holistic principle 'on an analogy with our own [human] causality' (page 57).

Such an interpretation brings to light the difference between a machine and a living thing. The parts of a machine fulfil the designer's purpose and the machine is completely knowable in terms of its parts. The living organism, on the other hand, understood only by analogy, is never completely known. It is not a machine. In that way the claim that man can be identified with a robot is refuted.

Following Kant, the mind apart from the brain is not accepted as an object for scientific enquiry which leads to an *ethical* interpretation: man is a subject, endowed with personal freedom and with responsibility. An existential philosophy is chosen to clarify the tenets of psychotherapy and of human life in general. Conscience is affirmed. The role of the therapist consists in facing the patient with the demands of his conscience. 'In the encounter with the therapist the patient is made aware of his struggle for freedom and authenticity' (page 160). Faith can be restored for those whose lives had been threatened by lack of meaning. The lack of this faith is at the root of the appalling state of the mental health of Western man. This is revealed by a recent survey conducted by the American Institute of Mental Health: one in every five Americans has a recognisable mental disorder, 13.1 million suffer from anxiety, 10 million from alcohol and drug abuse, 9.4 million from depression. These are severe disorders. Another study, carried out in the 1950s found that up to 80% 'had some mild level of impairment'. [1] Although drug addiction has not reached the same level in Great Britain as in America, depression, suicide and attempted suicide are very prevalent, and 'some 30 per cent or so of the population... present with chronic or recurrent symptoms of emotional stress and tension [and] ... 28 per cent of the children [in a disturbed family] have a poor outlook'. [2] Scientific psychiatry has no answer to this problem. The answer will be indicated in chapter 3 entitled 'Medicine and Ethics'.

NOTES

[1]   Science 1984; 226:324 and Report in 'Polling for Mental Health',
      Time, October 15, 1984.
[2]   Ryle, Anthony, 1967, *Neurosis in the Ordinary Family*, London:
      Tavistock, pp. 128, 88.

Acknowledgements

I should like to thank Mr David Horowitz for his help in the formulation of my views and Professor David Jenkins, Bishop of Durham, for his constructive criticisms.

'Where do I grasp you, boundless Nature?'
Goethe, Faust I.

Introduction

Medicine purports to be a scientific empirical discipline based strictly on observation. Doctors in the main believe that they carry on their practice without employing any general theory or philosophy, either in an overt or implicit way. It is the purpose of the present book to disprove this accepted view and to show that there is indeed a philosophy underlying every medical practice, moreover that there are a variety of philosophies, concurrently held in the medical profession, and that the differences between them lead to different forms of treatment. In what follows an attempt will be made to understand these fundamental philosophies and to comprehend their relations to the resulting practices, to ascertain the nature of the theories on which medicine is based and to investigate their scope and their limitations: in other words to look at medical theory from a philosophical point of view.

Medical science shares the characteristics of natural science, its language is the language of universals, the individual unique person is conceived as a particular example of a universal aspect of nature. The wholeness of his personality is split up into parts which are made into the material for scientific investigation and treatment, the main division being into body and mind, each of which is treated by a special branch of science, the body by biology and its sub-sciences, the mind by psychology.

The task for the biologist and the medical psychologist is to explain the phenomena which he has isolated. He assumes that they are the result of influences which have affected the material of his study. This assumption is the presupposition of determinism which can be formulated in a general way as follows: 'Every event A is so connected with a later event B that, given A, B must occur [1]'.

In the scientific explanation, an account is given *how* the event A is connected with the event B, what *mechanism* is involved. 'Mechanism implies the ignoring of the omnipresent individuality of the real and the imposition upon it of an abstract law which determines every case indifferently from the outside [2]'.

The matter whose mechanisms are studied by the medical scientist is the material which composes the body and the material which constitutes the psyche. In order to obtain a view of the method of medical

xix

science, let us envisage the investigation and treatment of a patient suffering from duodenal ulcer.

The diagnosis which classifies this man as a sufferer from the disease of duodenal ulcer abstracts from the wholeness of his unique personality. Although his subjective feeling of pain is taken into consideration as pointing to the presence of an objective lesion and although his feeling of anxiety is noted as a significant factor, the medical scientist as a scientist is not concerned with personal experience but with findings, with signs and symptoms of a disease.

The deterministic framework of mechanistic materialism poses the following question: what factors have caused the state of health A to be followed by the state B of disease? Although it was the whole man who was well and it is the whole man who is now ill, as the illness is a duodenal ulcer, the medical scientist abstracts from the rest of the personality and is concerned only with this particular part. He does not know *the* cause of this condition, but he isolates a number of factors which are involved: the ulcer, a defect in the lining of the duodenum, is associated in many cases with a discharge of highly acid stomach juice which enters into the duodenum, causing local damage. Apart from hypersecretion there is increased motility of the stomach due to over-activity of the vagus nerve. The disease, investigated from an epidemiological point of view, is very common in Great Britain (ten per cent of men are estimated to suffer from gastric or duodenal ulcer at some time of their lives, duodenal ulcer being in certain parts more common than gastric ulcer) and in certain other countries, but very uncommon in some parts of the globe. As the bearers of certain blood groups are more liable to the disease than those of other blood groups, a genetic factor plays a part.

The treatment is symptomatic: for duodenal ulcer there is no specific drug available, but there are drugs which diminish the secretion of gastric juice, which decrease the motility of the stomach and which neutralize the acid of the stomach or tend to suppress its secretion. All these drugs are used, giving some relief in many cases.

The effect of emotional factors is taken into consideration as such feelings as anger and resentment are known to lead to increased acid secretion and to hypermotility of the stomach. A variety of approaches is available to deal with the emotional disturbance: drugs are used which quieten the brain and in so doing the mind, or psychological treatment is employed. The Freudian school derives its conception of duodenal (and gastric) ulcer from the instinctual general theory: the patient is said to be orally frustrated, hungry for love. The hunger is supposed to cause the excess of secretion in the stomach which is associated with this condition. As he is not conscious of this mechanism, the patient requires psycho-analysis to work through this conflict.

The treatment by psycho-analysis differs from the other treatments which have been mentioned. The Freudian approach is not specifically directed against the particular illness, but the illness is interpreted as an expression of a general instinctual disturbance. The treatment is, however, as deterministic-mechanistic as the other forms of therapy, since the patient is taken to be the bearer of instinctual libido which is the material for the treatment, and which is supposed to undergo certain changes which constitute various mechanisms.

So far only *one* philosophy has been described with its clinical applications: the philosophy of mechanistic materialism. There is an alternative to this basic philosophical approach, leading to different forms of treatment.

The alternative view does not analyse and isolate phenomena, but starts from the whole person. Using Smuts's term, it can be called 'holistic', concerned with wholeness. The assumption is that health depends on the obedience to 'natural' laws, to certain ways of using body and mind, and that a deviation from the natural conditions, illness, is liable to occur, not just in one part but in many parts. As the medical scientist has not been trained to think in terms of wholeness, he is liable to miss the holistic approach, especially in the field of bodily disease where the scientific method is highly developed.

The patient suffering from duodenal ulcer can be treated on holistic lines. T. L. Cleave has pointed the way to such treatment and to the prevention of ulcers in the stomach and duodenum and, with the same approach, of other most prevalent conditions such as paradontal disease and caries, diabetes and coronary disease.

T. L. Cleave's approach is dietetic. With regard to ulcers in the stomach and the duodenum, dietetic treatment has been intensively studied and, according to the medical scientist, is not helpful. Milk diets, high protein regimes, high carbohydrate feeds have all been tried and without success. All these diets follow the analytical-specific approach of mechanistic materialism. T. L. Cleave is concerned with what is natural and not natural, with wholesomeness and unwholesomeness. He finds support for his views from the incidence of the disease which has been stressed. According to him, ulcers in the stomach and the duodenum (and the other diseases which have been mentioned) occur when people eat refined carbohydrates, i.e. white flour and sugar. In his book, *Peptic Ulcer* [3] he gives the evidence for his hypothesis: in countries where people live on unrefined products, on 'natural' diets, the disease is practically unknown. According to him, the rise of the consumption of sugar, an undoubted fact in countries like Great Britain, runs parallel with the rise of the disease. As further support for his thesis, he quotes the case of soldiers in the German army who during the second world war were forced to abstain from refined carbohydrates and had to eat coarse bread. Peptic ulcer which had been a common condition amongst the troops became very rare [4].

T. L. Cleave stresses not only the part played by unnatural processed carbohydrates, but also by the unnatural habit of eating without hunger. He blames the taking of unnecessary routine meals from the nursery onwards throughout life, often for conventional reasons, for the adoption of the unnatural eating-pattern [5].

The role of emotions enters into eating and over-eating. People use foods, especially the sweet foods which Cleave condemns, to satisfy emotional cravings. In a state of anxiety, the stomach is in fact not fit to digest food, and, as Cleave has pointed out, fasting is the correct treatment [6].

The holistic approach can be supported by a mechanistic argument: Cleave provides this argument by maintaining that the refining process deprives the grain of its natural protein which buffers the acid secreted by the stomach. In addition, he considers the absence of fibre in the processed foods to lead to imperfect mastication and thus to insufficient impregnation with saliva and to increased speed of emptying of the stomach, all factors which interfere with proper digestion. Thus health or wholeness is taken to depend on natural conditions which allow the mechanisms of normal and healthy functioning to take place, and a deviation from such conditions is made responsible for illness with its abnormal mechanisms.

F. Avery Jones, a specialist in digestive illnesses, has supported Cleave in his approach [7] and has agreed that Cleave's view 'is important not only in relation to ulcer but possibly to many other conditions as well, more even than he himself has postulated [8]'. R. Doll, Director of the Statistical Unit of the Medical Research Council and a Teacher in Medical Statistics and Epidemiology at the University College Hospital Medical School in London, has agreed that T. L. Cleave's and G. D. Campbell's 'observations . . . may provide clues to the causation of the common diseases of European civilization [9]'.

T. L. Cleave's book *Peptic Ulcer* was published in 1962 and *Diabetes, Coronorary Thrombosis and the Saccharine Disease* by

T. L. Cleave and G. D. Campbell was published in 1966; therefore the holistic view expressed in these publications has had sufficient time to influence the thoughts of medical scientists. It is impossible to predict the future, but it is possible to state the condition on which the acceptance of the views depends; the acceptance of the holistic view which is the philosophical underlying idea.

The holistic view is not new and previous presentations of it have not led to its acceptance, because of the prejudice against it, which may well not have been a conscious bias. For instance, Sir Robert McCarrison, a former Director of Research on Nutrition in India, expressed the same opinion on the role of unnatural foods in the production of disease which Cleave and Campbell hold, in his Cantor Lectures in 1936 [10]. Sir Robert McCarrison quoted gastric and duodenal ulcer as a disease due to faulty diet and prevalent among people who eat the wrong food (fifty-eight times more common in one part of India than in another [11]). In order to prove his thesis, McCarrison carried out experiments on rats, feeding one group on wholewheat flour, chapatties, butter, whole milk, raw fresh vegetables and fresh meat with bone, and the other group on white bread, margarine, tinned meat, boiled vegetables, tinned jam, tea, sugar with a little milk. The first group 'was fed on a diet similar to that used by the Sikhs' (who are healthy); 'the other on a diet such as is commonly used by the poorer classes in England. . . . The experiment was continued for 187 days, or for a period which would correspond to about sixteen years in man [12]'. The result of the experiment was as follows: 'Disease in the lungs was much commoner in the group fed on the poorer class Britisher's diet; gastro-intestinal disease . . . was frequent in this group, while that receiving the Sikh diet was free from it [13]'.

The difference between McCarrison's and Cleave's statements lies in the fact that McCarrison described the effects of diets which were deficient in minerals and vitamins apart from containing an excess of refined carbohydrates, whereas Cleave has investigated the results of consuing refined carbohydrates and has excluded other factors. Both McCarrison and Cleave stress the value of whole cereal grains.

McCarrison went further in his holistic view than Cleave does: he included the importance of the condition of the soil; he said: 'We found in India that foodstuffs grown on soil manured with farmyard manure were of higher nutritive quality than those grown on the same soil when manured with chemical manure [14]'. Disease in man and animals was related to wrong food and wrong food was related to wrong soil [15].

The full implementation of the holistic principle with regard to growing and preparing food for millions of civilized men raises many technical problems which cannot be discussed in this book. The practical importance of the principle is evident, but its acceptance by the medical scientist depends on his attitude towards the holistic approach. The theoretical implications of this approach need clarification, and the relationship to the mechanistic materialistic approach of science must be investigated. A further task consists in the elucidation of the holistic treatment of the mind. Here too, abnormal functioning may be prevented or helped by considering the normal conditions.

Whether we follow the philosophy of mechanistic materialism or of holism, the individual person is understood as the result of forces which determine his physical and mental make-up. A philosophical enquiry must go beyond the framework of determinism. It must consider the person as a free individual agent. Returning to the example of the sufferer from duodenal ulcer, this man must be approached by his doctor as a person who is facing the disabilities of his illness and the danger to his life which it brings about. The task of coping with any sickness as part of life is a moral task. The experience of life with all its vicissitudes is different for everybody. The doctor has to be aware of the particular subjective worlds in which his patients live and has to meet them in their worlds as persons, trying to help them in their struggle. The following enquiry will include the subjective and ethical sides of medical practice. The enquiry will start with a consideration of the two philosophies of medicine, mechanistic materialism and holism.

NOTES

[1] B. Blanchard, *The Case for Determinism* in *Determinism and Freedom in the Age of Modern Science*, Collier Books, New York, N.Y., 1961, p. 20.

[2] R. G. Collingwood, *Speculum Mentis or The Map of Knowledge*, Oxford at the Clarendon Press, 1924, p. 166.

[3] Publ. John Wright & Son, Bristol 1962.

[4] See *Diabetes, Coronary Thrombosis and the Saccharine Disease*, Bristol, John Wright & Sons, 1966, p. 96.

[5] ibid, p. 101.

[6] ibid, p. 102.

[7] Foreword to T. L. Cleave's book, *Peptic Ulcer*.

[8] ibid.

[9] Foreword to their book *Diabetes, Coronary Thrombosis and the Saccharine Disease*, Bristol, John Wright & Sons, 1966.

[10] Reprinted under the title *Nutrition and National Health* and published by Faber & Faber, London in 1944.

[11] ibid, p. 25.

[12] ibid, p. 24.

[13] ibid.

[14] ibid, p. 12.

[15] The significance of the holistic treatment of the soil is evident from the publications of the Soil Association, see their journal *Mother Earth*. Registered Office: New Bells Farm, Haughley, Suffolk.

CHAPTER I

Two Philosophies of Medicine

The Philosophy of Mechanistic Materialism

'The essence of materialism, its assertion of an indifferently self-identical substrate behind the variety of empirical fact, is unchanged whether this substrate is called matter, energy, or space-time. Materialism ... a logical phenomenon, it is the indifference of the abstract universal to its own particulars [1]'. Materialism is a form of idealism, a theory about the nature of the universe and mechanism gives an account of the changes within the assumed substrates, of the 'laws' of nature.

The scientist is engaged in observing nature, in empirical study of details and is apt to attribute to the material which he studies the status of universal essence. The field of the physicist (and chemist) has assumed this role. It is a field in which the scientific endeavour of formulating laws has been most successful and in which prediction of the sequence of events has been achieved. Certain biologists and medical scientists have accepted the dogma of physicalism.

MONISTIC PHYSICO-CHEMICAL MATERIALISM

As Collingwood has pointed out, materialism can be based on the assumption of an all-pervading energy instead of a universal material substrate. Biophysics makes use of such approach and identifies changes within the cells of living organisms with physical processes which involve the exchange of electrons between neighbouring groups of atoms. Such exchanges either give off energy or require energy. Biophysics have standardized the electron volt unit which is required for such exchanges: a very small amount of energy, about one billionth of the amount which is required to move two steel sewing pins one inch.

The energy is quantized, i.e. it is needed in packets. The application of the energy principle to medical science consists in explaining illness as an energy block preventing an exchange of energy between molecules; treatment would consist in removing such a block. According to this conception, man and other living things are merely a condensation of energy.

The concept of energy does not, however, allow biologists to account for the great variety of phenomena. Although chemistry is considered to be part of physics, the different compositions of chemical molecules offer a better explanation for biological phenomena; thus biochemistry as distinct from biophysics serves as the basis of much of biological theory.

Living organisms are composed of the same molecules which are the elements of inert matter. The processes which occur in the bodies of plants and animals are chemical processes. Oxidation plays a vital part in physiology, and biological oxidation is chemical oxidation consisting in the attachment of an oxygen atom to a substance which can be represented by a chemical structural formula.

The secrets of life are unravelled by the isolation of material chemical substances. An example is the discovery of the carrier of hereditary characteristics, the gene: deoxyribonucleic acid (DNA). The mechanistic materialist, basing his arguments on biophysical and biochemical research, holds that all biological phenomena can be explained in physico-chemical terms.

A mechanistic-materialistic explanation cannot ignore the difference between living and non-living things: the former have a marked tendency to maintain themselves as wholes by means of regulatory processes, whereas the latter lack such tendency. The maintenance of wholeness, the holistic principle, mentioned in the Introduction, implies a teleological explanation, which is denied by the mechanistic materialist who recognizes only independent, isolated parts and their relationships which enable him to apply the deterministic formula, quoted in the Introduction: 'Every event A is so connected with a later event B that, given A, B must occur [2]'.

The mechanistic materialist claims that teleological explanations can be translated into non-teleological equivalents. E. Nagel investigated this claim and we shall follow his argument [3]. The two types of explanations were characterized by Nagel as follows: 'teleological explanations focus attention on the culminations and products of specific processes, and in particular upon the contribution of various parts of a system to the maintenance of its global properties or modes of behaviour. They view the operations of things from the perspective of certain selected "wholes" or integrated systems to which things belong; and they are therefore concerned with characteristics of the parts of such wholes, only insofar as those traits of the parts are relevant to the various complex features or activities assumed to be distinctive of those wholes. Non-teleological explanations, on the other hand, direct attention primarily to the conditions under which specified processes are initiated or persist, and to the factors upon which the continued manifestations of certain inclusive traits of a system are contingent. They seek to exhibit the integrated behaviours of complex systems as the resultant of more elementary factors, frequently identified as constituent parts of those systems; and they are therefore concerned with traits of complex wholes almost exclusively to the extent that these traits are dependent on assumed characteristics of the elementary factors. In brief, the difference between teleological and non-teleological explanations . . . is one of emphasis and perspective in formulation [4]'.

The term 'system' requires a further elucidation. The chance of translating teleological, holistic explanations, used in biology, into non-teleological explanations, preferred in the physical sciences, depends on the possibility of expressing the principles of the biological system in terms of those of the physical system.

Nagel explained the difference in the two types of system. The living organism is a hierarchical system, the systems of inert matter are not. A cat, for example, exhibits the following hierarchy: the whole cat, its heart, its heart muscle, the cells composing the heart muscle, the atoms and molecules and the physico-chemical processes affecting them. The system 'cat' is a teleological system, an organic unity and it is impossible to deduce the functioning of this living organism from the physico-chemical laws of the atoms and molecules, i.e. from the lowest level of the hierarchy. Biology is thus not reducible to the physical sciences. Therefore a holistic approach is essential in biology [5].

The wholeness of a living organism like the human being (and of a mammal in general) consists of mind as well as body. In the behaviour of such beings, mental features such as will and emotions (for instance fear or anger) are clearly expressed. Monistic mechanistic materialism derives the mental features also from the physico-chemical constitution, i.e. denies their existence as mental features. In other words, this form of materialism denies the existence of psychology as well as of biology, reducing the phenomena of both sciences to the physical sciences.

In the total mechanistic-materialistic approach, the mind is replaced by the brain and the whole body (including the brain) is identified with a machine. Such a robot is explained by an application of chemical and physical laws, without teleological explanations.

The machine obviously works according to the laws of the physical sciences and certain modern machines are holistic: self-regulating and self-maintaining, having feed-back devices in them and self-control built in. Examples are engines constructed with governors, thermostats, automatic aeroplane pilots and radar-controlled anti-aircraft firing devices. Such machines are homeostats: self-maintaining systems, 'so organized that they are able to interchange with their surroundings without merging with them. One of the features of a homeostat is the presence of detectors that indicate tendencies of imbalance within it and set in motion actions that tend to correct them [6] '. The homeostat is therefore a set of physical events which responds to its surroundings in the appropriate manner according to the information it receives. ' "Information" may be defined as the feature of certain physical events in the communication channels of a homeostatic system that allows selection among a number of possible responses. The physical events in the channels are called "signals", and they transmit information in a "code". A code is thus essentially a set of physical events among which the appropriate members are selected to represent any given change in the surroundings. Encoding is the process of selecting the appropriate signals to represent any given change. Decoding is the action of an effector producing some operation on the environment that appropriately relates to the change encoded by the given signals [7] '.

The author of these definitions is an eminent biologist, J. Z. Young. He applies the machine concept of the homeostat to the living organism and the 'physical events' are for him the physiological phenomena which maintain or regulate the whole body of an animal or of man. Young has studied the holistic processes in the octopus and has drawn attention to the regulatory functions of nerve cells in respect of muscle fibres. He assumes that the nerve cells have a code which enables them to effect the appropriate muscular contractions. The muscle fibres, on their parts, have to 'decode' the transmitted information, contracting according to the signal which they have received from the nerve [8].

The brain plays a central part in Young's field of research. He uses the 'language' of computers to account for the cerebral phenomena and relates biology to physics by explaining physiological events (neural and muscular events for instance) in engineering terms, and he incorporates the field of psychology with physics by arguing: 'calculating machines and brains both think [9] '.

The last quotation requires careful analysis, for it is doubly misleading. The assertion that brains think appears to be obvious. To accept this assertion as a fact would, however, mean that the mind has lost its independence. As will be explained later on, such a view is unacceptable. What we are prepared to admit is that the mind thinks and that it needs for this activity the brain. This formulation preserves the mental field but admits that it is dependent on the physical (cerebral) sphere.

Certain modern philosophers argue that machines have minds like human beings. As a result of such a point of view, we find the following titles amongst philosophical papers: 'Could Machines Perceive? [10]' 'Can a Machine be Conscious? [11]' 'Discussion: Thinking and Machines [12].'

Robots differ from human beings in several respects. One difference can be formulated by referring to E. Nagel's distinction of biological and physico-chemical systems: the elements composing the former are not known in physico-chemical terms, but elements constituting the latter are so known. Therefore the mechanism of the machine can be explained completely with the aid of physical and chemical laws and the living organism cannot be reduced to the level of a machine and to the laws which govern the activities of machines. The neglect of the difference in the composition of robots and human beings has important consequences: the specific teleological behaviour of living organisms is denied, as it was by Rosenbluth, Wiener and Bigelow in their paper 'Behavior, Purpose and Teleology [13]' in which we read the following statement: 'Teleological behavior thus becomes synonymous with behavior controlled by negative feed-back [14]', and the consequences of such confusion become evident in the following passage, taken from a paper by Rosenbluth and Wiener: 'We believe that man and other animals are like machines from a scientific point of view because we believe that the *only* (italics mine) fruitful methods for the study of human and animal behavior are the methods applicable to the behavior of mechanical objects as well. . . . As objects of scientific enquiry, humans do not differ from machines [15]'.

While there is no doubt that humans do differ from machines in vital and basic ways, and while psychological and biological teleology cannot be legitimately denied, an *analogy* of psychical and biological phenomena with inert physical phenomena can be accepted.

The Model in Physico-chemical Materialism

Analogies are expressed by means of *models* which explain certain features of the particular phenomena which are unfamiliar and are made familiar by the model [16]. The model simplifies a complex phenomenon and thus makes it more intelligible, it has a 'heuristic' function [17], but it leaves features, not covered by the analogy, unexplained. The heart, for instance, can be explained analogically as a pump: this model accounts for the mechanical action of the heart, propelling the blood into the arteries, but it takes no account of the histological and biochemical features.

By selecting one particular feature of the phenomenon which is in need of explanation, for instance the motility of the heart muscle, the model takes on the characteristics of a metaphor and acts as a lens. 'The metaphor selects, emphasises, suppresses, and organises features of the principal subject by implying statements about it that normally apply to the subsidiary subject [18]'. The selective quality of the metaphor 'allows some things to pass, disallows others. It organises the things which pass through it in some sort of systematic fashion. It selects some things over others. It *rearranges* things [19]'. The metaphor thus acts as a *filter*.

The model is different in its structure from the thing which it explains, and the terms 'analogy' and 'metaphor' imply that there is a difference between the two objects. Inverted commas signify that we use the language of analogy. The situation becomes complicated in the case of the brain; for here the model is to explain not only physiological but also psychological functioning.

One important function of the brain is memory, which enables its bearer to learn. J. Z. Young defines the term 'memory' in the sense in which engineers employ it: as 'the unit within which the record is stored [20]'. (Young points out that the record of the single event is not necessarily localized in one place, but may be carried by changes at many points in a multi-channel system [21].)

If the language of engineering is used to account for biological and psychological phenomena, the analogous character of this language gets lost. The memory of the computer is not the memory of the living cell, and the memory of the mind is different from the memory of the machine and from that of the brain although it is dependent on the biological memory. Young maintains that 'we shall advance in our study of memory only when we recognize that the brain is the computer of a homeostat and that the memory provides part of the information by which the homeostat selects correct responses [22]'. Young uses the computer as a model in order to illustrate the memory function of the brain; when he speaks of 'information' in the two systems, he refers to physiological phenomena in the case of the brain, to psychological ones in the case of the mind. The computer as a piece of machinery obtains its 'information' from the human being who has programmed it; this information is therefore no part of the machine, although it has a machine-equivalent in the stored information.

The term 'model' does not only refer to a physical structure: it also refers to a theory. J. W. Swanson has defined the theoretical model as follows: 'An original theory or field of investigation T_1 has been delimited and probed in preliminary fashion, but remains incomplete and contains gaps. Subsequently, a second more developed theory T_2, which we call "the model", is found to share certain structural similarities with T_1, which we call either "the interpretation" or "the theory" .... If the structure of all the relations of the model T_2 carry over in this fashion (viz. of analogy) to the interpretation T_1, then one says that there exists an isomorphism of structure between model and interpretation [23]'.

For the application of the model theory, it is therefore necessary to be in the possession of two theories, sufficiently known in their respective structures so that one theory can serve as the model for the other. The example quoted by Swanson is the model of the atom and its model the theory of the planets circulating around the sun.

If we accept Swanson's definition, it is clear that we would require adequate knowledge of the theory of the computer and of the theory of the brain if we were justified in making the former theory a model for the latter. Such knowledge would have to reveal such closeness of the theories that the structure of the one could be used as the image for the structure of the other.

A leading article in the *British Medical Journal* has examined the relationship between the computer and the brain [24]. The writer of this article comes to the conclusion that although the brain and the computer have electrical discharges in common, this fact does not entitle us to consider the brain as working like a computer. 'The living cell has its own laws and the nervous impulse no counterpart. . . . The electrical impulse is an abstraction from nervous activity; it is not itself nervous activity. Similarly, the electrical computing machine embodies an abstraction from the multifarious activities of the brain [25]'. We are therefore not justified in taking a mechanistic physico-chemical theory as the model for a biological theory, and even less justified in identifying the psychological memory with the biological memory. As was pointed out earlier on, we are at present ignorant with regard to the detailed functioning of biological structure, a fact which J. Z. Young freely admits [26, 27].

As biological phenomena not only differ from non-living phenomena, but as the details of biological dynamics are not known at present, a biological all-embracing theory cannot be illuminated by means of a physico-chemical theory. Thus physicalism fails in biology not only in its direct application to the biological phenomena, but also in its indirect application by means of analogous reasoning. Physicalism fails also in the explanation of psychological phenomena in general which, it assumes, are a manifestation of physiological phenomena.

To refuse a mechanistic materialistic explanation of biology and psychology on the basis of the physical sciences does not prevent the biologist or psychologist from explaining *individual* phenomena by means of analogies taken from the physical sciences. Such explanations do not involve a general physicalistic claim. Examples are the model of the pump to explain the action of the heart and the model of the lock and key to illustrate the relationship of the antigen and the antibody. In the field of psychology analogies with physical processes are commonly expressed in the figurative language which is used in this discipline. Emotions are said to be 'suppressed', 'inhibited', 'sublimated' and instincts 'perverted'. The use of such analogies does not necessarily imply an acceptance of a general libidinal theory based on principles of physicalism; such analogies serve to illustrate a certain mechanism without necessarily referring to an overall theory.

MONISTIC BIOLOGICAL MECHANISTIC MATERIALISM

A mechanistic-materialistic approach is not restricted to physicalism; 'the indifferently self-identical substrate behind the variety of empirical fact' (Collingwood) can be identified as an all-pervading *biological* substance. The present generation of biologists does not make such an assumption, but a former generation did. P. B. Medawar refers to such substrate in his paper *A Biological Retrospect* [28]. He mentions 'Hopkins's famous aphorism from the British Association meeting of 1913, that the life of the cell is "the expression of a particular dynamic equilibrium in a polyphasic system [29]"', and refers to 'the doctrine of "protoplasm"' as the idea of 'a fragile colloidal slime, a sort of biological ether permeating otherwise inanimate structures [30]'. Such 'colloidal conception' of life 'allowed for heterogeneity [31]' and thus is an illustration of Collingwood's notion of materialism.

While modern biologists do not derive the individual phenomena from a common substrate and do not conceive the mechanisms in the living organism as changes within such substrate which can be studied in isolation, certain psychologists follow a biological mechanistic-material-istic course. They make the nerve cell and its biological activities the basis of psychic life. These psychologists are *behaviourists*.

Pavlovian psychology is basic to behaviourism and to the theory of behaviour therapy. Pavlov reduced all psychological phenomena to physiological cerebral phenomena. His physiology was concerned with the response of the cortex to stimuli which excite or inhibit the activity of the cells.

Automatic, neurological phenomena are isolated as the uncondi-tioned and the conditioned reflex. Dogs are used to prove the theory; the sight of meat is the unconditioned stimulus which produces saliva-tion, and the ringing of a bell, associated with the unconditioned stimulus as the conditioned stimulus, in time, also produces salivation. Salivation is a reflex which thus results as an unconditioned or con-ditioned reflex from the respective stimuli.

In the Pavlovian scheme seeing and hearing are only physiological processes and are deprived of their subjective experiential meanings. The nervous system is conceived as an aggregate, the whole living being, animal or man, a biological apparatus. Thus the principle of deter-minism, 'every event A is so connected with a later event B that, given A, B must occur' is put into operation. Reflexology provides the mechanism within the physiological, neural substrate.

Pavlov's dogs were trained to respond to stimuli. Human beings can also be trained and can be made to perform in an automatic, deter-ministic way as performing animals. The behaviourist Watson applied Pavlov's theory to man and asked: 'Give us your babies, and we will place them in our laboratories, study their squirmings and condition them into artists, bricklayers, physicians, teachers, street cleaners, university professors and what not [32] '.

J. Wolpe, an outstanding exponent of behaviour therapy, works on the assumption of the causal relationship between stimulus and re-sponse and assumes the existence of an underlying neural correlate. He explains the effects of his therapy as 'molecular' or 'molar' responses, i.e. as changes in small units or as the gross resultant of these [33] .

Wolpe bases his psychotherapy on a learning theory, which is of the event A — event B type, A being a stimulus, B the response to the stimu-lus. Wolpe's definition of learning is as follows: 'learning may be said to have occurred if a response has been evoked in temporal contiguity with a given sensory stimulus and it is subsequently found that the stimulus can evoke the response although it could not have done so before [34] '. The substrate which underlies the learning process is according to Wolpe the nervous system, in particular the conductivity between neurones in anatomical apposition [35]. Neurotic behaviour is interpreted as the result of certain stimuli and must be treated by 'unlearning'.

It is important to realize not only that the human being or the animal is reduced to the vehicle of a neural response arising from a neural substrate, but that the environment is also reduced to being just a stimulus arising from an indifferent ground. Erwin Straus has drawn attention to the artificiality of such experiments and has criticized their environmental setting as follows: 'The experimental arrangement imposes from the outset a constriction of the situation. . . . Stimuli that are perfectly standard in the animal's natural environment are first carefully eliminated from the laboratory. Subsequently, they are re-introduced. But this time they are allowed to appear only at the moment preceding the feeding. In this way, the precedents of the experiment create a neutral situation. By a kind of impoverishment, the environment is so restricted that ordinary processes and common stimuli may eventually assume abnormal prominence [36]'. The two-fold impoverishment is the price which behaviourists have to pay for their brand of mechanistic materialism.

The process of learning which plays such a large part in Wolpe's theory reveals the restriction of the behaviouristic approach. Straus has criticized the behaviouristic learning theory for its narrowness. To him, the experience with its total involvement of the animal or man is the essence in learning. Satisfaction or pain are the vital experiences; these are converted by the behaviourist into individual stimuli influencing individual nerve cells.

In fact, as Straus has pointed out, Pavlov's dogs only respond to the unconditioned and conditioned stimulus in a completely artificial laboratory environment. If a cat entered the laboratory, the dog would not respond in the correct manner. The dog would not respond either to the sight of the meat or its associated sound if it was not hungry. Thus the state of the whole dog is decisive and the environment is normally incorporated in the whole situation, as an animal looks upon it as a *goal*, for instance the place where it finds its food to satisfy its hunger.

Learning also involves purposiveness, i.e. attention of the whole animal. As Straus points out, the animal learns to find its food in the laboratory or outside and learns to avoid making mistakes in trial runs [36].

The human being is also involved as a whole person in the learning experience. It is not the 'stimulus' which causes the neurotic anxiety but the meaning or significance of the situation. Wolpe's own examples bear out the fallacy of his theory. He quotes as examples of phobias the case of a man who developed phobic reactions to roughly dressed men after he had been assaulted by hooligans and the case of a woman who suffered from anxiety at defecation after a painful rectal examination [38]. Both these patients had been subjected to a total frightening situation and not to a molar or molecular stimulus. Their state cannot be explained on the basis of their neural cells. In their response, their total personalities are involved. (Behaviour therapy may help them to face their situation, but this success cannot be explained on the strength of the behaviouristic theory).

NOTES

[1] R. C. Collingwood, *Speculum Mentis or The Map of Knowledge*, Oxford at the Clarendon Press, 1924, p. 167.
[2] B. Blanshard, *The Case for Determinism in the Age of Modern Science*, Collier Books, New York, 1961, p. 20.
[3] *The Structure of Science, Problems in the Logic of Scientific Explanation*, London, Routledge & Kegan Paul, 1961, chapter 12.
[4] ibid, p. 422.
[5] The holistic school affirms that its approach will *always* be essential in biology; Nagel does not accept this statement and points out that future research may make it possible to apply physico-chemical explanations to vital systems. According to him, such possibility depends on the detailed knowledge of the physico-chemical composition of a living organism and of the forces acting between the elements of the lowest hierarchical level, knowledge which is at present not available.
[6] J. Z. Young, *A Model of the Brain*, Oxford, Clarendon Press, 1964, p. 3.
[7] ibid, p. 20.
[9] ibid, p. 49.
[9] ibid, p. 6.
[10] By Alan Gauld, *British Journal for the Philosophy of Science*, May 1966, vol. 17, part 1, pp. 44-58.
[11] Dennis Thompson, *British Journal for the Philosophy of Science*, 1966, vol. 16, no. 5 and a reply to his paper by Robert J. Clack in the same Journal in vol. 17, no. 3, pp. 232-4.
[12] By A. D. Ritchie, W. Mays, in *Philosophy*, July 1957, pp. 258-61.
[13] *Philosophy of Science*, publ. by The Williams and Wilkins Co., Baltimore, Maryland, Jan. 1943, vol. 10, no. 1.

[14] ibid, p. 18.

[15] 'Purposeful and Non-Purposeful Behaviour', *Philosophy of Science*, vol. 17, no. 6, Oct. 1950, p. 325.

[16] See D. W. Theobald, 'Models and Method', *Philosophy*, July 1964, vol. 39, no. 149, pp. 261, 262.

[17] ibid, p. 264.

[18] Max Black, *Models and Metaphors: Studies in Language and Philosophy*, Cornell University Press 1962, pp. 44-45.

[19] J. W. Swanson, 'On Models', *Brit. J. Phil. Sci.* (1966), vol. 17, no. 4, p. 306.

[20] *The Memory System of the Brain*, Oxford University Press, 1966, p. 17.

[21] ibid, pp. 21, 22.

[22] ibid, p. 17.

[23] 'On Models', *British Journal for the Philosophy of Science*, vol. 17, no. 4, Feb. 1967, pp. 298, 299.

[24] 'Mind Machine and Man', *British Medical Journal*, 25 June 1949.

[25] ibid, p. 1129.

[26] In the Philosophy of Science the term 'model' is not only used to describe explanations by means of physical structures or by theories. The term is also used to denote a pattern of an explanation for a type of phenomenon, i.e. a model in this sense represents a certain theory under which certain empirical observations can be subsumed; such models are called 'deductive' or 'implicational' models. See for instance Morton Beckner, *Aspects of Explanation in Biological Theory*, chapter 14 in *Philosophy of Science Today*, ed. S. Morgenbesser, Basic Books, Inc., New York and London, 1967. As the discussion is concerned with the application of mechanistic-materialistic principles to biological and psychological phenomena, we are not interested in the relationship of the empirical material to its *own* theory, but in the relationship of one type of phenomenon to a *different* type of phenomenon and its theory, a relationship which is analogous.

[27] Rejecting the computer as a suitable model for the explanation of the functioning of the brain does not invalidate the use of the computer for analysing biological phenomena, for instance photomicrographs of chromosomes. In such cases, the computer simply carries out work which is otherwise carried out by a human being and the work can be done by the computer because a human being has programmed it. Thus the computer is simply used as a machine in its own right and not as a model to explain biological phenomena.

[28] Reprinted in *The Art of the Soluble*, Methuen & Co., London, 1967.

[29] ibid, p. 106.

[30] *The Art of the Soluble*, Methuen & Co., London, 1967, p. 105.

[31] ibid, p. 106.

[32] 'Behaviourism', by Watson, quoted in *Behaviourism*, Student Christian Movement Press, London 1930, p. 123.

[33] *Psychotherapy by Reciprocal Inhibition*, Stanford University Press, 1958, p. 4.

[34] 'Psychotherapy: The Nonscientific Heritage and the New Science', *Behaviour Research and Therapy*, Pergamon Press, Oxford, London, New York, Paris, vol. 1, no. 1, May 1963, p. 26.

[35] 'Learning versus Lesions as the Basis of Neurotic Behaviour', *American Journal of Psychology*, vol. 112, no. 11, May 1956, p. 926.

[36] *The Primary World of Senses*, The Free Press of Glencoe, Collier-MacMillan Ltd., London, 1963, p. 83.

[37] ibid, p. 137.

[38] 'Learning versus Lesion as the Basis of Neurotic Behaviour', *American Journal of Psychology*, vol. 112, no. 11, May 1956, p. 926.

PART II
The Philosophy of Holism

The behaviourist theory cannot account for higher animal and human behaviour because of the narrowness of its two basic concepts, learning and reflex, which both express the deterministic pattern of stimulus-response. Human and animal mammal behaviour is a manifestation of total individuals endowed with minds which are motivated by goals and living in a world of meaningful experiences.

Medical science depends on a deterministic framework and postulates a 'self-identical substrate behind the variety of empirical fact'. By conceiving bodily or psychic matter to answer to a stimulus in deterministic manner, the medical scientist can develop theories which enable him to understand and to treat patients scientifically.

We saw that the machine can serve as a model for living organisms or parts of it, but that living matter is fundamentally different from non-living machine matter, hence the holistic, teleological element resists the scientist's purge. It is therefore necessary to accept this element and to see how it can be accommodated *within* the domain of scientific endeavour.

The totality of the personality, its wholeness, is affirmed by the philosophy of holism. Smuts coined the word 'holism' 'to designate this whole-ward tendency in Nature, this fundamental feature of "wholes" in the universe [1]'. Smuts held that holism was 'an ultimate feature of the world [2]', manifest in the inorganic world in atoms and molecules, in the organic world in the plants and animals and in the human personality comprising body, mind and spirit and its creations. Holism according to Smuts is 'disclosed' as 'the motive force behind Evolution [3]'. 'Conceived as an absolute principle, holism is a counterpart to materialism to the indifferently identical substrate behind the variety of empirical fact' (Collingwood), providing the form to these substrates. Materialism and holism emerge as the complementary determining principles which are both essential for the explanation of the phenomena which exist in the universe. The holistic force is teleological. 'Teleology is purposiveness, and "purposiveness" is a special form of that unified action which ... means a correlation and unification of

16

actions towards an end, whether this is consciously conceived or apprehended or not [4]'.

When discussing the philosophy of mechanistic materialism, we met the problem of the teleological explanation in biology. We found that such explanations were autonomous and could not be translated into non-teleological explanations, which meant that biological organisms could not be explained merely according to the laws of the physical sciences. The machine, constructed with the aid of the physical sciences, played a prominent part in the discussion. As a homeostat, a self-regulating and self-maintaining physical system, the machine was accepted as a model of the holistic living thing, but the analogous character of the model, we found, did not justify the claim that organic wholes *are* machines, According to Smuts, the holistic principle is manifest in living organisms and the mind, and in a simpler form in the atom and the molecule. The role of holism in these structures will now be examined.

HOLISM IN PHYSICS AND BIOLOGY

Smuts' view that the atom and the molecule are holistic structures produced by nature is shared by many people. The view is erroneous. The mistake arises through a study of atomic models which are pictured as holistic structures consisting of a central nucleus and a certain number of electrons moving around the nucleus as the planets move around the sun. Such models are constructs which scientists have invented for theoretical reasons. In nature, non-living matter does not behave in this orderly holistic fashion. 'The planetary electrons very rarely behave in any way like planets. . . . It is never possible to perceive anything which could, by the widest stretching of language, be called order, system or organization [5]'. Molecules, found in nature, also lack in order or organization. The theoretical knowledge of the atomic structure is fruitful for the acquisition of knowledge of chemical properties of inorganic matter, but the laws of chemistry and physics alone cannot account for the holistic object which is called a machine. 'To say that a thing is a mere machine is to say that it is more fully determined than any structure which results only from the unaided action of Matter on Matter [6]'. As Kapp has pointed out, machines serve purposes to men, and as structures, designed to serve a purpose, they are determined teleologically as well as physico-chemically, the telos being human purpose.

The machine depends on human telos in its design, construction and maintenance. To some degree the self-maintaining machines which have been likened to self-maintaining living organisms are independent of man after they have been put into operation by man, but they soon need overhauls, therefore their independence is short-lived. With regard to computers, they are constructed in such a way that the human telos can programme their actions; they are thus completely dependent in their performance on human telos. The difference between machines and living things thus lies not only in the elements which compose these structures, but also in their teleologies: the machine depends on human purpose, its matter itself showing no innate purposefulness, whereas living things are independent of human purpose and contain teleology within themselves.

The acknowledgement of the teleological principle as a factor which is additional to the laws of physics and chemistry provides further insight into the question, discussed by Nagel, which was investigated earlier, namely whether vital organisms will ever be explainable entirely according to the laws of the physical sciences. We must answer the question in the negative sense, as the laws of the physical sciences cannot provide the additional teleological principle. As Kapp put it, 'it is not enough for atoms of hydrogen, carbon, nitrogen and oxygen to be put together in any way which may conform to the laws of physics and chemistry. Among all the possible ways which would meet this first [physico-chemical] requirement only those are permitted in the organic world which also meet the second [the organic-teleological] requirement. If this does not happen the result is not even remotely like an organism [7]'.

As the teleological principle is responsible for bringing about the essential features in living things, medical scientists whose task is to account for the functioning of the human body in health and disease, concentrate their attention on the manifestations of this principle.

The purpose of the heart is to pump blood into the arteries, veins and capillaries to bring the blood into contact with all the tissues of the body, the purpose of the lungs is to supply the body with oxygen and to remove carbon dioxide, etc. The finer structures of an organ serve its purpose and thus the purpose of the whole organism. The heart and the arteries require muscles to function and therefore the muscle fibres answer the purpose of the body, the histological construction of the lungs is necessary for the exchange of gases to take place. In these and in innumerable other examples does the medical scientist see the principle of teleology, the holistic principle, at work.

Tracing the regulative, holistic arrangement, the physiologist isolates

centres which regulate such vital functions as breathing or the
beating of the heart. These centres are located in the central nervous
system.

An important aspect of holism is the principle of constancy of the
main constituents of the body, the composition of the blood, the body
temperature, the oxygen supply, etc. W. B. Cannon coined the term
'homeostasis' to designate this holistic feature. In cases of illness, the
homeostatic mechanisms may be temporarily disturbed; the treatment
aims at the restoration of the equilibrium, and the body itself tends to
work towards the establishment of the whole through its ability to heal
a wound, to compensate for lost functions by parts of the body taking
over the role of those parts which are out of action (one kidney for
instance can work for two).

Homeostasis also applies to metabolism, to the building up of bodily
material and its decomposition. Physiologists have discovered that the
metabolism is regulated by hormones and by enzymes which work
according to the principle of feed-back inhibition which means that the
production of a certain substance is inhibited when a certain amount of
this substance has accumulated in the cell. Furthermore, there is an
homeostatic interplay between the metabolism of such essential substances as fats and sugars.

The acquisition of immunity against harmful invaders is a teleological process. The organism protects itself through the formation of
antibodies which combine with the foreign substances and thus render
them inactive. The holistic process can go wrong and illness can be
explained in that way. Sir MacFarlane Burnet postulates that the body
can distinguish normally between 'the self and not-self [8]', auto-
immune diseases are explained as a failure in this differentiation.

Cannon's book is entitled *The Wisdom of the Body* and the dis-
crimination between self and not-self must be counted as a confirmation of such wisdom, which implies the ability to act in a purposeful,
holistic manner.

Medical scientists are not content with a general holistic conception
of the living organism. They study the ways in which the body achieves
its task of maintaining itself as a whole, they study the holistic mechanisms in detail. They employ for such investigations the holistic
structure which the chemist has made the basis of his science, the
structure of the atom and the molecule, and they make also use of
human purposefulness which we found is evident in the construction of
the holistic machine. We shall first discuss the application of atomic
holism and then the employment of human teleology.

In his paper, *A Biological Retrospect*, P. F. Medawar discusses different levels of biological study: 'We have molecular biologists, whose ambition is to interpret biological performances explicitly in terms of molecular structures; we have cellular biologists, biologists who work at the level of whole organisms (the domain of classical physiology), and biologists who study communities or societies of organisms [9]'. In the first two planes a part (the molecule and the cell) and in the other two levels the wholeness (of the organism and of different communities forming a whole population) is fundamental. Medawar illustrates his thesis by mentioning geneticists and divides them according to the four planes of study into 'molecular and cellular geneticists' and into geneticists in Mendel's sense, and population geneticists [10]'. The holistic orientation is obvious in the third and the fourth plane, but it is also evident in the first two, as the molecule and the cell are holistic structures, although different, the former exhibiting the theoretical, invented purposefulness of chemistry and the latter the natural inherent purposefulness of biological phenomena.

Biologists explain the holistic function of the biological system with reference to the molecular structure of one of its constituents, the gene, which has earlier on been identified as deoxyribonucleic acid (DNA). The DNA molecules contain certain parts, called bases; it has been found that the sequence of bases in the DNA molecule determines the structure of particular protein molecules which are specific for each organism. Thus the particular configuration of the DNA molecule determines the holistic (or in cases of disease) the unholistic nature of the particular organism. According to Sir MacFarlane Burnet, an autoimmune disease is the result of a genetic fault.

In the investigation of how the gene determines the characteristics of an organism, the biologist assumes the existence of a teleological principle which is conceived to be of the same kind as human teleology. In the discussion on mechanistic materialism we met this form of teleology. It was manifest in the machine, for instance in the homeostat and in the computer. An understanding of the nature of the machine has led to the conclusion that the teleological principle in the machine cannot be considered as part of inanimate nature, but must be recognized as a manifestation of the human mind which constructs and programmes machines, for instance the computer. We accepted the principle of analogy in order to account for the phenomenon of self-regulation which is characteristic of machines with feed-back mechanisms and for all living organisms, but we disagreed that living organisms *are* machines.

In the science of genetics, we meet the language of human purpose-fulness: the genes are said to contain information which is required by the cell to reproduce itself, and this information is in a coded form, embodied in the molecular structure of the gene.

The code, we learnt, was defined by J. Z. Young as 'a set of physical events among which the appropriate members are selected to represent any given change in the surroundings', and 'information' was defined by the same author as 'the feature of certain physical events in the communication channels of a homeostatic system that allows selection among a number of possible responses [11]'. Thus a code and the information which it transmits were interpreted as parts of a physical system which was said to be part of the science of engineering.

As all products of engineering require for their understanding the acknowledgement of human teleology, we cannot accept the code and its information just as parts of inanimate nature.

Molecular biologists use the term 'code' to account for the relation-ship which exists between two structures, the structure of the nucleic acid molecule in the cell nucleus and of the particular cell protein molecule. They assume that these two structures use forms of languages in coded form and that the code enables the biologist to understand how the short language of the nucleic acid controls the long language of the protein. 'Protein synthesis takes place on the comparatively large intracellular structures known as ribosomes. These bodies travel along the chain of messenger RNA [12]', the letters standing for ribonucleic acid. Thus, although molecules, they are also messages [13].

It is confusing to read that 'genes are not ... models [14]' and that the words 'messengers', 'messages', 'language' etc. — all obviously refer-ring to human teleological activities — are printed without the inverted commas when they refer to the activities of molecules in biological structures.

As the molecular biologists have been successful in the application of these notions, as their experiments, based on human teleology, have yielded spectacular results, the use of such teleology must be accepted. Its nature must be ascertained: biological molecular structures behave in a way which shows the characteristics of human purposefulness without being in the possession of a mind which can think purpose-fully. The notion of purpose is thus an essential notion to account for the particular phenomena; together with the notion of the material substrate it enables the scientist to explain deterministically the pattern of these biological phenomena.

HOLISM IN MEDICAL PSYCHOLOGY

Like the body, the mind tends to maintain itself. It stands up to strains as does the body and is treated on the assumption that it can regain its equilibrium when disturbed. Mental health like physical health involves the recognition of a holistic force within the mind.

The holistic structure of the mind may be said to be less evident than is the holistic configuration of the body. Conflicts are unholistic and are an integral part of mental life. Different schools of psychological medicine differ in their holistic interpretations.

The discussion of mechanistic materialism brought to light the views of behaviourism, which denies the existence of a mind apart from the body. Behaviouristic claims were refuted.

Psycho-analysis is a system which grants independence to the mind. It views the mental structure holistically and interprets neurotic illness as the result of a failure to maintain its wholeness. O. Fenichel, a Freudian, described the theory as follows: 'All neurotic phenomena are based on insufficiencies of the normal control apparatus. They can be understood as involuntary emergency discharges that supplant the normal ones. The insufficiency can be brought about in two ways. One way is through an increase in the influx of stimuli: too much excitation enters the mental apparatus in a given unit of time and cannot be mastered; such experiences are called traumatic. The other way is through a previous blocking or decrease of discharges which has produced a damming up of tensions within the organism so that normal excitations now operate relatively like traumatic ones [15]'.

Freud assumed that instinctual energy strives for discharge and he postulated as a regulative force the ego which defends the mind against being flooded with instinctual energy. These defensive efforts are found manifest in neurotic symptoms.

When evaluating the significance of the Freudian holistic apparatus, it is important to realize that the efforts to prevent a breakdown of the mind as a whole are not the efforts of an individual person, but of the psychic control apparatus of which he is said to be a bearer (just as he is a bearer of a biological control apparatus). The theory is deterministic, assuming certain forces which result in the maintenance of the whole or in its breakdown.

According to psycho-analysts, the individual is further determined by the social group of which he is a member. He is exposed to the holistic and to the unholistic forces of this group. 'There are disrupting and integrating forces in every group. In social groups, the latter are encouraged and the former denied, so that the movement is steadily towards greater integration. Social groups do disrupt, nevertheless, because the suppressed disrupting forces start an underground movement of their own [16]'.

Freud was convinced that the wholeness of the individual mind and of the human community was threatened by the instinct of aggression and self-destruction.

In the Freudian scheme, the individual and the community are thus seen as subject to holistic and unholistic forces; their existence is derived from the observation which Freud and his followers have made on their patients. He named the two opposing forces the life instinct, eros, and the death instinct, and he assumed that mental phenomena are composed of a mixture of these fundamental tendencies.

The holistic tendency is traced in its manifestation of object seeking, and mechanisms of the establishment of emotional ties between persons are postulated: identification with the love object which may be followed by introjection. The unholistic tendency is seen in sadistic and masochistic activities which are taken to depend on the punitive attitude of the super-ego.

The psychic activities are studied as involving tension and abolition of tension through discharge of libidinal energy. The getting rid of tension leads to a state of constancy, and this state has been deduced from the principle of homeostasis which we met as an expression of holism in biology. 'Homeostasis is, as a principle, at the root of all instinctual behavior; the frequent "counterhomeostatic" behavior must be explained as a secondary complication, imposed upon the organism by external forces [17]'.

Freudian psychology is instinctual; instincts are biological forces, thus the deterministic material-holistic conception follows the lines of biological reasoning.

Neo-Freudians have abandoned the biological orientation and have replaced it by emphasis on object relations. The holistic state is then the state of a strong ego which can maintain good object-relations. The unholistic state of the patient has been characterized by H. Guntrip as follows: 'We may now summarize the position in which we find our patients, one which is more marked and recognizable in proportion as they are seriously ill. The menaced ego is like a hare hunted by hounds; whichever way it turns it runs into a different danger. If the total self, weakened by a basic Regressed Ego, takes refuge in good objects it feels claustrophobically suffocated; if it chooses bad objects, it risks schizophrenic disintegration; if it compromises by an ambivalent relationship with an object which is seen as both good and bad, it heads for guilt and depressive paralysis, and if in despair it takes flight from all object-relationships, it runs into loss of itself by de-personalization, by feeling emptied and reduced to nothing by having nothing with which to maintain any living experience [18]'. The holistic state is envisaged by Guntrip, when he goes on to say: 'The only hope lies in seeing through and overcoming the fears of loss of independence in good object-relations and the chance of this is what the psychotherapist offers [19]'. The formulation by Guntrip is as deterministic as the Freudian formulation. The individual patient's ego is a bearer of the ego which Guntrip postulates as the victim of conflicts, of being split, of having been deprived of energy which is locked away in the unconscious, an ego which has suffered strains in childhood which it relives in adult life. All these and other vicissitudes are those of the ego in general. The teleology is that of an object which has the tendency within itself to gain its wholeness in relation to other objects.

THE HOLISTIC PRINCIPLE

Psychotherapists and physicians as well as surgeons who treat patients for physical ailments rely on the holistic response from the mind or the body. The stimulation whether by word or by drug or any other physical agent is intended to call forth a whole-making result, which is the same sort of result which is present when mind or body answer to the 'normal' stimuli which arise from within it or which arrive from without. The centres of regulations within the central nervous system and the effectors which are connected with these centres in the different organs all point to the existence of a holistic principle as such which is manifest throughout the body and mind.

To any unprejudiced observer who witnesses the vital significance of the holistic principle in all forms of medical practice and also in the realm of medical theory, it must seem strange that this principle is not recognized. Although it is implied in such concepts as homeostasis, equilibrium or health, it is never named overtly. The reason for this neglect is historical.

The assertion of a teleological principle present in living organisms (especially in living bodies) used to be made by a group of thinkers who called themselves 'vitalists'. They were opposed by another group, 'the mechanists' who held that the living thing can be explained according to the laws of the physical sciences. The vitalists assumed that a living force, an entelechy (i.e. something which had a telos in itself) was an 'agent at work in morphogenesis', i.e. in the creation of the individual out of its parts [20]. This 'agent' was also 'required' to arrange the material units on which heredity depended [21], its presence was further 'proved' by the integrated behaviour of body and mind in human activity [22].

The mechanist denies the need for such assumption; to him research is mechanistic, the living organism is treated like a machine; the vitalist points out that the machine requires a machinist, which is the vital, teleological principle.

By postulating the need for a teleological principle, evident in biological and psychological phenomena, we appear to have joined the ranks of the vitalists. Such allegiance would ostracize us in the world of scientific thinkers. Driesch's entelechy seems out of date. In the field of heredity, geneticists have discovered the mechanism of the arrangement of the hereditary material units and embryology is linked with genetics. As P. B. Medawar has pointed out, 'embryonic development at the level of molecular differentiation must be ... an acting-out of genetically encoded instructions [23]'.

We must reply to the mechanists that the language of the geneticists uses the principle of teleology; the terms 'information', 'instruction', 'code' and others are not part of the vocabulary of the physical sciences. These teleological notions are essential for the explanation of phenomena met in biology, as the teleological principle is essential in the explanation of psychic phenomena.

The quarrel between mechanists and vitalists has died down, the assertion of opposed doctrines is fruitless. Scientists discover more and more mechanisms, which are, however, subject to the 'vitalistic' (i.e. biological or human teleological) holistic principle.

THE HOLISTIC PRINCIPLE IN MEDICAL PRACTICE

(a) Bodily Illness

The researches, based on the 'mechanistic' approach lead to the discovery of specific phenomena in the body and the mind, and the treatment of physical and mental illness consists in the application of these researches. In fact, to a large extent, medicine has become a technical affair like engineering. The different parts of the body are treated by different specialists and another group of specialists treats the mind. The future of medical and surgical treatment promises to be an enormous extension of specific measures, as more details of the composition of the body and of its different individual functions are discovered. The treatment by specific drugs is an example of this approach, drugs which also affect the brain and which thus are successful in mental illness.

The neglect of the holistic principle is wrong. It is not sufficient to take it for granted in the specific approach, to admit that the body must respond as a whole to surgical and pharmacological measures, the importance of the holistic principle must never be ignored which has been the case as a result of the advances in the detailed study.

The mechanistic approach has led to advances in therapy as in the treatment of infectious diseases; it has enabled surgeons to remove diseased parts such as inflamed gall bladders and appendices and thus to cure patients; it has also led to prevention of illness through immunization, but it has not solved the problem of degenerative diseases and cancer. True, many scientists are engaged in the study of these conditions, and their exact mechanism may become known which would lead to effective specific treatment. Doctors, however, cannot just wait for the result of such research, they have to act *now*; they miss opportunities for effective treatment by neglecting the teleological principle.

The principle of wholeness is the principle of health. Medicine has largely become the treatment of sickness because of its attention to detailed disease processes. The prevention of illness (which is obviously better than its cure) depends on the proper functioning of the whole body (and mind) on the conditions under which health is possible, and health is a matter of wholeness. The state of disease can also be influenced by holistic treatment, i.e. by improving the physiological conditions under which the person lives.

The example of duodenal ulcer which was quoted in the Introduction illustrates the importance of the holistic approach. This very common condition cannot be treated successfully, as its cause is not known, and as no specific drug for its cure is available. Dietetic treatment, based on the isolation of food articles — high protein, high carbohydrate regimes for instance — have been tried in vain; their prescriptions arise from the attempt to find a specific factor which will cure the ulcer. Specific, palliative measures, such as prescriptions of alkalis, are obviously not satisfactory, as they are not curative.

T. L. Cleave, we saw, claimed that his approach succeeded where other measures failed. Cleave has been supported by a specialist in digestive disorders and by a teacher in medical statistics and epidemiology. The approach considers the natural conditions, i.e. those factors which the body requires for health. The refined carbohydrates were found to be the main cause of disease. Wrong living does not only cause peptic ulcers, it is also responsible for such diverse conditions as para-dontal disease and tooth caries, diabetes and coronary heart disease. R. Doll has admitted that the observations, based on this approach 'may provide clues to the causation of the common diseases of European civilization [24]'. Wrong living causes a general state of disease, and right living prevents such a state or can lead back to health.

The dogmatic use of 'right' and 'wrong' must be avoided. Civilized life entails enduring unnatural 'wrong' conditions; urban populations especially do not lead healthy natural lives, and their foods have to be stored, which involves the use of artificial measures. The holistic principle cannot be fulfilled in the ideal way. It can only be realized as far as it is possible under the existing circumstances. The school of *natural therapy* treats patients according to the holistic principle and advocates healthy living as far as it is possible in order to avoid illness.

The holistic approach of natural therapy consists in the use of stimuli to which the *whole* body responds. Dietetic measures play a prominent part; they are not primarily prescribed for the treatment of individual diseases, but for the treatment of individual sick people. Diet can be a stimulus and not just a supply of caloric units. Dietetic stimuli are graded according to intensity; a fast on water is the most drastic measure; prescribing of fruit juices makes the treatment less drastic. Further steps are the introduction of raw vegetables, cooked vegetables, milk protein and wholemeal bread. Such treatment is indicated in acute and in chronic illnesses, but the illness is not the decisive factor; what matters is whether a particular patient will respond to the diet. The literature of natural therapy gives many illustrations of such regimes.

Apart from diet, natural therapy consists in the use of stimuli to the skin: hot and cold water, air and sun; all these stimuli are also graded according to the needs of the particular patient and his ability to respond.

Muscular exercise is encouraged and properly graded by natural therapists. There is no doubt that many modern people suffer from lack of exercise. The significance of this lack has recently been evaluated with regard to coronary heart disease, and a number of authors consider lack of exercise to be an important factor in this condition (muscular exercise increases the work of the heart muscle considerably and thus the blood circulation in this muscle). Muscular exercise also affects the action of endocrine glands, respiration and metabolism. Physical exercise thus affects the whole person. Apart from its physiological importance, it has also undoubted psychological effects [25, 26].

(b) Mental (emotional) Illness

As the concept of wholeness is not applicable to the same extent to the psyche as it is applicable to the body, the holistic approach to emotional or mental illness is also less clear-cut in this sphere than in the sphere of bodily health. It is, however, possible to distinguish the unspecific holistic conception from the specific one.

The distinction of the two conceptions gets blurred in the field of analytical psychotherapy. On the one hand, the emphasis on the total person requiring treatment and receiving psycho-analysis makes this form of therapy holistic. The emphasis on the role of the ego as the bearer of the holistic element supports this view. On the other hand, the libidinal character of the treatment singles out one aspect of the human psyche and is therefore not holistic.

Psycho-analysts are very emphatic that their form of therapy is not a form of suggestion. Suggestion to them means that the therapist does nothing to change the faulty dynamic conditions, that he does not deal with the conflict which underlies the emotional illness, that he suppresses the symptoms which are a manifestation of the conflict.

Suggestion can, however, be used in an unspecific manner and not as a means of removing symptoms. Used in that way, suggestion treatment relies on the mind's ability to achieve a better state of integration; it appeals to the self-healing, holistic mental tendencies.

HOLISTIC SUGGESTION

Suggestion is practised by all doctors, whatever the treatment, whether it is a medicine to swallow or an injection or an operation. The idea accompanying all these prescriptions is: this will help you. The doctor's personality conveys the general suggestion that the patient will get better. This optimism forms an integral part of medical practice. The patient needs such assurance to counteract his own fear of disease and death and the implied suggestion that he will not recover.

Apart from the using of suggestion as an integral and generally unconscious element in all medicines, it can be practised deliberately as a form of psychotherapy. Coué made it into a system of healing and described his method in a book which became famous [27]. The general formula which has become associated with his name is 'every day, in every way, I am getting better [28]'. The effect of this formula

is explained by Coué's conception of the mind as a 'mysterious laboratory' which he thought belonged to the 'subconscious self' and which
'instantaneously translated (the suggestion) into an active living
force [29]'.

Charles Baudouin also examined the theory of suggestion and the
underlying conception of mental life, and like Coué looked upon the
subconscious as the part of the mind which is concerned in this treatment [30]. The suggestion itself represents an idea, and the subconscious mind takes it up and realizes it in practice. The work of the
unconscious (or the subconscious in the words of Coué and Baudouin)
goes on continuously even during sleep and the following phases can be
distinguished in this process: the idea is conceived by the mind, then
the unconscious starts to work on it, and finally a change of the mind
takes place. Such classification of phases has practical consequences, as
it allows a therapist to act accordingly. It is also important to understand to what types of suggestions the mind is open. Baudouin distinguished three classes: firstly 'representative' suggestions. These
include sensations, mental images, judgements and opinions which are
presented to a person and incorporated into his mind. The second
group embraces 'affective' suggestions. Here we have ideas of a sensation of pleasure or pain which tends to be realized by the patient. The
negative suggestions with their negative effects have to be particularly
remembered. Baudouin quotes the common example of a child which
has fallen down. If the mother says: 'It doesn't hurt', the child does feel
little if any pain, whereas, if she says: 'You have hurt yourself terribly',
the child immediately feels a great deal of pain. The example shows
that it is the idea of feeling pain which is the operative factor and not
the degree of actual injury. Baudouin goes so far as to say that we are
sad because we weep — sadness having been suggested to us — and not
that we weep because we are sad. Amongst the negative feelings, fear
and anger are particularly powerful suggestive influences.

The third group comprises 'active or motor' suggestions. Movement
often follows as the result of the first two types of suggestion, but the
idea of motion is itself a strong suggestive power which produces
movement directly. Habits of eating, drinking, and various additions are
cited under this heading. Organic processes in the body such as the
course of tubercular infections as well as so-called functional diseases
without any organic basis can be influenced by suggesting a different
form of behaviour of the particular organs affected. The importance for
medicine is obvious.

HOLISTIC ENVIRONMENTAL TREATMENTS

As natural therapy allows the body to effect a cure by enabling the various organs to function under more favourable conditions, so certain forms of psychotherapy lead to recovery from mental disturbances by placing the patient under more congenial circumstances. These are so devised as to offer the patient opportunities for expressing his own holistic, i.e. self-healing, potentialities.

A break from work and from the routine of life at home is one of the most usual ways of finding strength to cope with life. A holiday often acts more on the mind than on the body, and the change of surroundings constitutes a stimulus as well as a relief. The new activities, whether they are mountaineering, swimming or golfing provide a contrast with life at home and at work. On return from the holiday the old troubles can be faced anew and often seem much less formidable. The holiday has released the inherent holistic power and is thus a form of holistic treatment of the body and mind.

In cases of emotional illness, the holiday is often an escape from troubles and has no lasting beneficial effect; it is too haphazard. Psychiatrists may *plan*, however, a change of surroundings and adapt such a change to the requirements of the particular patient. This is *situational* treatment [31]. Situational treatment is used in mental hospitals as occupational therapy.

'Occupational therapy provides a controlled environment for personalities not ready to meet the demands of everyday life. Throughout, the control can be gradually lifted at the right pace, so preparing the patient with a positive attitude, and with an initiative to take responsibility in preparation for a full, useful life [32]'. Life itself enables people to develop their personalities; occupational therapy thus represents a form of life and it shares the holistic effect with life in general.

The patient improves because the activities he undertakes draw him out of himself. This is particularly important in the case of withdrawn personalities, schizoids and schizophrenics who life in a world of delusions and fantasies [33].

Occupational treatment is not confined to the mental hospital. It has been realized that patients suffering from all sorts of physical diseases benefit from well-selected activities. This applies in particular to those patients who have a chronic disease which prevents them from pursuing their usual activities for a lengthy period. Tuberculosis is an example. A. Rollier, a pioneer in the use of sunlight for surgical tuberculosis, also employed occupational therapy for his patients [34]. A. Hill, a modern painter, has shown the beneficial effects which painting has in the case of tuberculosis of the lungs, and this has become accepted by physicians in charge of such cases [35].

Situational treatment is widely used in the case of disturbed children as *Play Therapy*. The children are provided with toys and other materials for play, such as sand and water [37].

Situational treatment of adults is beneficial because it brings the patient face to face with reality. This represents a challenge to his innate faculties of adjusting himself to the requirements of life. The same consideration has led to the development of a special branch of medical psychology, which is based on a complementary holistic relationship; the individual's desire and ability to integrate himself within a social whole, a community, on the one hand, and the latter's desire and ability to integrate the individual within its compass on the other. These general human factors operate in a special way in the case of the mentally sick: ordinary society tends to exclude them (because its members fear insane and emotionally disturbed people, as they remind them of their own mental instability and the most frightening possibility of losing their own mental balance). The patients, already unsure of their place in society, are made a great deal worse by the social stigma. Their need for company and reassurance is great, and is met by *social psychiatry*.

According to Thomas A. C. Rennie, social psychiatry 'seeks to determine the significant facts in family and society which affects adaptation (or which can be clearly defined as of etiological importance) as revealed through the studies of individuals or groups functioning in their natural setting. It concerns itself not only with the mentally ill but with the problems of adjustment of all persons in society toward a better understanding of how people adapt and what forces tend to damage or enhance their adaptive capacities. . . . Social psychiatry is therefore the study of etiology and dynamics of persons seen in their total environmental setting [37]'.

The family is the first natural holistic force in a person's life. The neurotic who has failed to integrate himself into his family and who has not succeeded in establishing the right relationships with its members, is given a further chance through the treatment. He finds a father or mother figure in the psychotherapist. The occupational therapist may play the role of a sister [38]. The other patients and the staff of the hospital represent the wider society, the general social milieu. In order to mobilize the holistic forces, patients are placed into groups or into Social Therapeutic Clubs [39].

Holistic medicine relies on whole-making tendencies, in the case of social psychiatry, the whole is a community of people. The question has been raised as to whether neurotics and psychotics do not make each other worse when grouped together, but experience shows that this is not the case. S. H. Foulkes explains the beneficial effects of such treatment by pointing out that the group brings out in the patient the common good and tends to make him lose the neurotic element which acts in an anti-social way. 'Neurotic symptoms disappear into the common pool as soon as they become communicable, and the individual ingredient is now free for group-syntonic, socially acceptable employment. That is the reason why neurotic behaviour tends to diminish in a Group and normal behaviour to be supported [40] '.

The group treatment of *children* requires special consideration. They are limited in their ability to express themselves verbally. Apart from the use of materials discussed already, the human factor is of the greatest importance for their development and in their treatment. The family is a natural group in which they express their love and hatred and in which they learn to become social beings.

S. R. Slavson has examined the factors which play a part in the treatment of children in groups. He has reorganized this to be a form of situational treatment and has pointed out the great possibilities which it has for the development and training of children and adolescents. He has found that integration is achieved 'by living in a therapeutic atmosphere and by corrective experiences and reactions [41] '. The children experience the group situation as a kind of family situation and clear themselves of their pent-up emotions in the 'catharsis'. This, Slavson holds, gives only temporary relief. He maintains that emotional maturity which is the aim of the treatment can only be achieved through insight and that the realistic situation of the group provides for this without analysis by the doctor.

The holistic forces of a therapeutic group or club, of the social situation, of suggestion which all affect the mind, or of unspecific dietetic treatment, hydro- and heliotherapy, air baths and physical exercise which affect the body, cannot be trusted implicitly. They can bring about health or prevent illness, but they may fail to do so. The unspecific approach is thus limited, and it is the duty of the therapist to assess each patient's condition and to apply specific measures, based on the mechanistic-materialistic approach, if necessary.

A person, suffering from mental illness, may require a drug to relieve depression; after such successful treatment, he will be even more likely to benefit from social holistic treatment. A heart which is failing may need strengthening with digitalis, and then the patient whose circulation has been improved by the drug may respond more fully to holistic natural therapy. The dogmatic holistic attitude has no place in medical practice.

As doctors are trained to think in terms of specific functions and parts, they are inclined to use the specific remedies which medical science has developed whenever a person is ill, at least bodily ill.

Some medical scientists have protested against the uncritical application of the specific-mechanistic principle, especially against the excessive prescription of drugs. They have pointed out that the abuse of drugs often leads to new illness. Sir Derrick Dunlop is one of these critics; he has stated that 'from 10 to 15% of patients in our general hospitals are suffering to a greater or lesser extent from our efforts to treat them — from iatrogenic diseases as they are called, or, more optimistically, from diseases due to medical progress [42]'. This author contrasts the efforts of medical scientists with Nature's own efforts. He considers Nature to tend to preserve a balance which is a holistic conception. Medical scientists upset this balance and often find their efforts directed at healing thwarted by nature: 'Our powers over nature in applied pharmacology', says Sir Derrick Dunlop, 'have extended so far that nature seems to have become retaliatory and is exacting a heavy retribution [43]'.

An iatrogenic disease may arise as the result of the application of a drug which was necessary to save a patient's life; for instance an antibiotic may have to be used in such a situation and may cause a serious state of unbalance of the normal microbial inhabitants in the intestinal canal. As the title of the paper by Sir Derrick Dunlop, *Use and Abuse of Drugs*, suggests, the author does, however, consider that iatrogenic disease is often avoidable.

Sir Derrick Dunlop quotes three reasons for the overprescribing of drugs: the demands from the public, the lack of time in medical practice which encourages doctors to prescribe medicine where a thorough examination would have led to a different form of treatment and 'the formidable and skilled promotion of drugs by the pharmaceutical houses [44]'. This list is not complete and leaves out the most fundamental factor: doctors have not been taught to consider first the natural, holistic approach before they interfere with the innate powers of healing. The public have accepted the attitude of the medical profession and expect the doctor to use modern powerful drugs. Science to them is a means of quick relief; hence the very excessive demand for hypnotics, sedatives, tranquillizers, analgesics, etc. and their equally very heavy supply.

The neglect of the holistic approach in medical practice arises therefore from a fault in medical and lay education. The individual practitioner and the individual patient suffer the consequences of the present-day form of medical science which tends to ignore the holistic principle. The neglect is more obvious in the field of bodily illness where the methods of natural therapy offer a clear first line of treatment; in the field of emotional or mental illness the situation is more complex, as a simple holistic approach is not always available (the mind not being a simple holistic system); such treatments as social therapy require special facilities which are not always available [45].

THE HOLISTIC PRINCIPLE AND THE MATERIAL SUBSTRATE

The scientist is inclined to ignore the holistic principle. His efforts are directed towards quantitative measurement, towards exactness. The vital principle strikes him as a force which eludes any such exact approach.

Driesch's conception of the 'entelechy', his term (borrowed from Aristotle) for the holistic force, illustrates the difficulty which the scientist experiences with regard to the acceptance of the holistic principle: entelechy was to Driesch 'an actual elementary agent or factor of Nature [46]'. Driesch had to find an answer to the questions how this 'agent' could influence the substrate on which it was supposed to work. He held that it was 'neither dependent on a spatial substance nor energy itself, nor creative of energy [47]', but that the entelechy controlled material systems and did so by suspending certain possibilities which caused the effects witnessed in organic phenomena [48].

The conception of an holistic agent and of the material on which this agent imposes its rule is scientifically unacceptable, as the agent cannot be measured and therefore the relationship to its field of action cannot be investigated.

While the concept of the holistic agent must be rejected, therapists rely on the presence of the holistic power in their patients overtly and implicitly. They cannot measure this power in units, but they attempt to gauge its strength. A surgeon for instance who envisages a major operation on a patient must assess this person's capacity to stand up to the strain of the operation, and he must therefore estimate his vitality,

his holistic power. Any doctor is concerned with the holistic recuper-
ative power of his patients.

The patient's vitality, his resistance against illness and his power to
recuperate from an illness, is not as a rule discussed in medical practice.
Instead, patients are subjected to detailed investigation; their blood is
examined for signs of anaemia or for the presence of an infection
somewhere in the body, their weight is taken and their state of nutrition is estimated – all such tests are considered relevant to estimate the
patient's 'vitality'. If a patient does not respond to a drug, given for
instance to combat an infection, the explanation is that the micro-
organisms, responsible for the infection, are not sensitive to the drug;
the explanation is thus not in terms of a lack of vitality. If he succumbs
to an infection, the medical scientist will find the explanation in the
absence of anti-body formation. Such an explanation still leaves the
question unanswered: why do the cells in the body which normally
produce antibodies fail to do so in this case? The medical scientist may
answer: because this patient had been weakened by a previous illness or
by age, in other words, the doctor would adduce a specific cause and
would not invoke the agent of the vital force.

The medical scientist should not deny the existence of a force which
is responsible for the existence and the operation of the various regulative and homeostatic mechanisms. As his approach is concerned with
the details of these mechanisms, he takes this force for granted. He does
not separate it from the material on which it exerts its power.

In the same way, the biologist does not separate the teleological
principle from the material which such a principle can be said to
govern. As J. H. Woodger has pointed out, 'to invoke entelechies as
agents at the point where the materialistic machinist gets into difficulties has not proved to be of any value from the methodological
standpoint because it is too successful, too general and gives us no light
upon the particular case. Entelechies are in just the same position as
energy when the latter is regarded as "the cause of changes in matter",
and such an appeal to imperceptibles is contrary to the present tendencies in scientific thought [49]'.

To the biologist, the concept of the holistic teleological entelechy is
unnecessary for his way of explaining living phenomena, to him the
concept is purely methodological. For the therapist, the concept stands
for an entity which he must not ignore. The recognition of the teleological factor makes a difference in his practice insofar as he avoids
any unnecessary interference with this principle.

Medical practice in its specific approach treats the parts in isolation;

in its unspecific approach it avoids such separation and trusts the holistic teleological principle, relying on the innate mechanisms which maintain life. The holistic approach is valid for the treatment of disease, but is even more important for its prevention, as, by considering the different aspects of the whole man, body and mind can function under conditions which tend to promote health.

Holism is a force which doctors trust when treating patients; holism is an attribute of bodies and minds, a regulative principle. Holism is a conception used by biologists like Sir MacFarlane Burnet who credits the organism with the ability to distinguish between self and not-self or like Cannon who ascribed to the body the wisdom of homeostatic mechanisms, holism is expressed in such concepts as the gene which is instrumental in giving a message and conveying information. Holism is postulated in the concept of the atom and the molecule, ideal structures, not present in nature, and holism is in the machine, a whole structure which owes its existence to man's purposeful thought. Holism stands for purposiveness, for teleology. Holism is related to the material of which the whole is composed, a material which consists of individual parts which medical scientists investigate. Scientific knowledge is knowledge of these parts and of their properties, of the constitution of cells, organs, their relation to one another and of their relation to other material parts such as drugs. In the organic wholes of body and mind the individual parts and their functions are related to the whole.

The whole body and the whole mind are themselves parts within the surrounding *milieu* and are subject to environmental forces. For instance, the food which is introduced into the body affects the whole body and a change of diet can profoundly affect vital functions. The individual mind is influenced by other minds with which it comes into contact, society is a large whole which determines the small wholes of its members. Thus the two philosophies of holism and mechanistic materialism are complementary, but their significance for medical science requires clarification.

The following problems arise: what is the relationship of the whole body to the whole mind, i.e. how can these wholes be related to the whole of the personality? What is the relationship of the biological or psychological whole to the abstract concepts which express the theory? Are observable biological and psychological phenomena holistic apart from being composed of certain elements which can be isolated and known? All these questions will be discussed in the next chapter.

NOTES

[1] *Holism and Evolution*, Third Edition, Macmillan & Co., London, 1936, p. 96.

[2] ibid, p. 97.

[3] ibid.

[4] ibid, p. 143.

[5] R. O. Kapp, *Science versus Materialism*, Methuen & Co., London, 1940, p. 170.

[6] ibid, p. 74.

[7] ibid, p. 87.

[8] See for instance his paper, 'The Mechanism of Immunity', *Scientific American*, January 1961, p. 5.

[9] ibid, p. 101.

[10] Sir MacFarlane Burnet, 'The Mechanism of Immunity', *Scientific American*, January 1961, p. 101.

[11] *A Model of the Brain*, Oxford, Clarendon Press, 1964, p. 20.

[12] F. H. C. Crick, 'The Genetic Code: III', *Scientific American*, October 1966, vol. 215, no. 4, p. 4.

[13] See P. B. Medawar, *The Art of the Soluble*, Methuen & Co., 1967, p. 100.

[14] ibid.

[15] *The Psychoanalytic Theory of Neurosis*, Norton & Co. Inc., New York and Kegan Paul, Trench, Trubner & Co., London, 1945, p. 19.

[16] S. H. Foulkes and E. J. Anthony, *Group Psychotherapy, The Psycho-analytic Approach*, Penguin Books, 1957, London, p. 209.

[17] O. Fenichel, *The Psychoanalytic Theory of Neurosis*, Norton & Co., Inc., New York and Kegan Paul, Trench, Trubner & Co., London, 1945, p. 13.

[18] *Personality Structure and Human Interaction*, The Hogarth Press and The Institute of Psycho-analysis, London, 1961, p. 439.

[19] ibid.

[20] H. Driesch, *The Problem of Individuality*, Macmillan & Co., London, 1914, p. 19.

[21] ibid, p. 23.

[22] ibid, pp. 23, 24-36.

[23] *The Art of the Soluble*, Methuen & Co., London, 1967, p. 57.

[24] Foreword to T. L. Cleave and G. D. Campbell, *Diabetes, Coronary Thrombosis and the Saccharine Disease*, Bristol, John Wright & Sons, 1966.

[25] J. V. G. A. Durnin has investigated claims of the benefit of exercise and counterclaims in *The Physiology of Human Survival*, edited by O. G. Edholm and A. L. Bacharach, 1965, Academic Press, London, New York in chapter 10; he distinguishes the subjective

from the objective value and confirms the beneficial effects of physical exercise in both respects.

[26] For an exposition of the principles of Natural Therapy, see E. K. Ledermann, *Natural Therapy*, 1953, Watts & Co., London.

[27] *My Method*, William Heinemann, Ltd., 1923.

[28] ibid, p. 26.

[29] ibid, p. 27.

[30] *Suggestion and Autosuggestion*, translated by Eden and Cedar Paul, Allen and Unwin, 2nd edition, 1924.

[31] See J. Bierer, 'Group Psychotherapy', *British Medical Journal*, 1942, I, pp. 214-16.

[32] K. M. Thompson, *Occupational Therapy, Modern Trends in Psychological Medicine*, Hoeber and Butterworth, 1948, p. 308.

[33] Art treatment plays a special part in freeing the emotional life and in allowing the patient to express his conflicts. Creative activity in the form of art is symbolic, and a patient may feel that his artistic work has liberated energy which results in a feeling of satisfaction. The therapist can interpret the picture or work of sculpture on analytical lines to the patient and thus raise unconscious material to his conscious mind. Such treatment would not be holistic according to the definition given.

[34] *The International Factory Clinic for the Treatment by Sun and Work of Indiginent Cases of 'Surgical' Tuberculosis*, by A. Rollier, Librairie Payot-Cie, Lausanne, Neuchatel, Geneve, Vevey, Montreux, Berne, 1929.

[35] *Art Versus Illness*, by A. Hill, Allen and Unwin, 1945.

[36] A playroom allows a child to live its life of fantasy. The therapist can use interpretations and thus confront the child with the unconscious feelings, for instance his hatred for his father played out in the hitting of the father doll. Through such interpretations which may not be necessary the treatment would lose its holistic character. The child can improve merely because of the therapeutic environment.

[37] Thomas A. C. Rennie, 'Social Psychiatry – A Definition', *International Journal of Social Psychiatry*, vol. 1, no. 1, pp. 12, 13.

[38] See paper by Inez Huntting, 'The Importance of Interaction between Patient and the Occupational Therapist', *American Journal of Occupational Therapy*, vol. 7, no. 3, May-June, 1953.

[39] The groups differ in size. In them and in the Clubs, the patient experiences social life in a sheltered form under conditions largely controlled by the therapist. The therapist can use the experience of the group situation as material for analysis or the members of the group can analyse each other's feelings and actions. In that case, the situational treatment of social psychiatry becomes non-holistic.

[40] *Introduction to Group-Analytic Psychotherapy, Studies in the Social Integration of Individuals and Groups*, Heinemann Medical Books Ltd., 1948, pp. 30 and 31.

[41] *Analytic Group Psychotherapy with Children, Adolescents and Adults*, Columbia University Press, New York, 1950, p. 12.

[42] 'Use and Abuse of Drugs', *British Medical Journal*, 21 August 1965, p. 439.

[43] ibid.

[44] ibid, p. 438.

[45] The measures of psychological holistic therapy do not arouse the same degree of opposition which doctors show against natural therapy which is almost exclusively practised by non-medical practitioners in Great Britain.

[46] *The Problem of Individuality*, Macmillan & Co., 1914, London, p. 33.

[47] ibid, p. 36,

[48] ibid, p. 39.

[49] *Biological Principles*, London, Kegan Paul, Trench, Trubner & Co.; New York, Harcourt, Brace & Co., 1929, p. 266.

CHAPTER II

Medicine and the 'Copernican Revolution' in Thought

Kantian Epistemology and Science

THE 'COPERNICAN REVOLUTION' IN THOUGHT

The philosophies of mechanistic materialism and of holism are theories about the nature of the universe and its features. They thus both exhibit a basic outlook which assumes that the world can be known as it is. This view forms the substance of the theory of knowledge, generally termed *naive realism*. Modern thinkers have tried to establish what they consider to be an alternative theory called *the theory of the sense-datum*. They think that they can avoid any reference to reality by confining themselves to what the scientist perceives by means of his senses. Many contemporary British and American philosophers would, however, admit that the sense-datum theory fails to be a really separate theory because what the theory presupposes is, in fact, identical with the assumption of naive realism: you cannot talk about perception without assuming the existence of objects which are perceived [1].

Mechanistic materialism and holism lead to an interpretation of the patient in terms of individual parts and cause-effect relations, and in terms of wholes and holistic forces respectively. As we have seen, the two ways of regarding phenomena are complementary and are both necessary to a balanced understanding. What remains to be considered, however, is the relationship between mechanistic materialism and holism, in particular how the parts are related to a whole. To answer this question, a clear understanding of the nature of wholeness is required. Although, according to Smuts, wholeness exists in the universe, it cannot be said to exist in the same way as do individual particles. The holistic force acts upon the parts and represents 'in' the organism the element of purpose leading to an integration of the different elements.

The assumption of purposeful activity without a personal Designer, however, presents a difficulty which, as we saw, the philosophy of holism cannot solve. In fact, this difficulty arises from the approach of naive realism itself which, because it considers the world to be knowable as such, makes metaphysical statements about the ontological structure of the universe.

A different philosophical approach is required to eliminate the difficulties presented by the theories we have examined. It has to throw light on the relationship between the principles of mechanistic materialism and holism, avoid the dogmatism of ontological metaphysics and at the same time accommodate both the deterministic principle of science and the principle of free will in ethics. Such an approach exists and was formulated by Immanuel Kant.

Where scientists and doctors concentrate on dividing up objects with which they are presented, into units, endowing these with the purposeful feature of wholeness, Kant turns his attention away from the objects and from the alleged principles of their integration to the foundations of the knowledge of these objects. This is a reversal of direction which amounts to a revolution in thought, and which Kant himself referred to as the 'Copernican Revolution'. Copernicus reversed the naive view that the stars revolved around the stationary earth and showed that the apparent movements of the stars were, in fact, due to the movements of the observer. Kant, similarly, explained the apparent characteristics of reality as the result of the processes which take place in the mind of the knower. The naive observer is equally unaware of either movement: the one which takes place in his mind when thinking as a scientist, and the other which his body performs when rotating on the earth around the sun [2].

What follows from the 'Copernican Revolution'? How does the mind build up a body of knowledge? In the Kantian outlook the objects of science lose their independence from the observer and become phenomena, i.e. appearances (to the mind). They do not lose their reality, however. In fact, it is the essence of Kant's theory of knowledge to accept the empirical objects as real and to bridge over from this reality to the world of knowledge. The bridge is signified by the term 'transcendental' which stands for 'the mode of our knowledge of objects in so far as this mode of knowledge is possible *a priori* [3] '. As objects of knowledge the phenomena bear the imprint of the scientist's mind.

In Kant's view the scientist perceives phenomena as occurring in space and time, and raises them to the status of knowledge by the use of certain *a priori* concepts ('categories of understanding') i.e. quantity, quality, relation and modality. I shall discuss in detail only one of the fundamental *a priori* concepts, namely, *causality*, which is a form of relatedness.

Science is concerned with the formulation of laws and rules which enable us to predict the course of events. The scientist discovers phenomena which he must conceive as being related to others in a fixed way. When undertaking research, the scientist makes the presupposition that the phenomena do not occur in an arbitrary, capricious manner; otherwise there would be no point in trying to make the scientific discoveries. Thus the scientist presupposes *necessity*. This is implied in the very concept of the cause. In Kant's view, causality is not to be sought in nature but in the mind; it is an *a priori* concept, essential for the creation of scientific knowledge.

Kant's concept of causality has been questioned because in modern physics a situation has arisen which appears to contradict the principle of causality. The physicist is unable to devise an experiment by which he can simultaneously fix the speed and the position of a single electron accurately. The reason for this fundamental uncertainty lies in the fact that the physicist 'can obtain knowledge of the internal state of the atom only by causing it to discharge a full quantum of radiation' . . . but 'the emission of a quantum of radiation is so atom-shaking an event that the whole motion of the atom is changed and the result is practically a new atom [4]'. Under these circumstances Sir James Jeans drew the following conclusion: 'It is futile to discuss whether the motion of the atom conforms to a causal law or not. The mere formulation of the law of causality presupposes the existence of an isolated objective system which an isolated observer can observe without disturbing it [5]'.

In the case of the single electron, it is thus impossible to formulate a causal law. Can the concept of causality be preserved under such circumstances? Jeans, himself, was aware of the problem. He agreed that the assumption of causality was an essential presupposition for the whole of science. Without it, science 'would seem to be left hanging in the air, with no justification for its existence, and no explanation of its success'. 'Yet', comments Jeans, 'the success is indisputable, and an explanation there must be [6]'.

He found the explanation in the fact that indeterminism is confined to the small-scale processes of nature and that even these 'indeterminate events are governed by statistical laws [7]'. In the realm where, in principle, observations can be carried out without altering the state of the observed object, 'nature is, to all appearances, strictly deterministic; like causes produce like effects. Thus the uniformity of nature is re-established [8]'. Hence the concept of causality can be applied even in those cases in which the chain of cause and effect cannot be demonstrated, and the Kantian view is vindicated. It accounts for the way in which the scientist's mind works: the phenomena of science are perceived in space and in time and are made into objects of knowledge by means of certain *a priori* concepts, causality being one of them.

SCIENCE AND METAPHYSICS

A central aspect of Kant's approach to the problem of knowledge is his distinction between metaphysical and scientific concepts and his delineation of the limits of the scientific realm.

Scientists are not free to invent any concepts. The criterion of the scientific character of a concept lies in its applicability to experience and, in particular, the experience of a single scientist concerned with a limited field of knowledge. Scientific concepts always refer to a limited field, to finiteness. Some scientific concepts, such as 'energy' or 'entropy' do not refer to an observable phenomenon directly and cannot themselves be perceived, but they refer to phenomena which can be perceived by a single observer.

Scientific theory makes no claim to absolute truth; on the contrary, it is only tentative. In fact, the hall-mark of a scientific theory is that it is possible to refute it. Refutability is an even more important feature of scientific theory than verification, as Popper has shown. With a broad enough basis practically everything can find confirmation, whereas the test of a scientific theory is that its basis must be small enough for the possibility of it failing to account for some phenomena. The refutability of a theory is an expression of the fact that it is limited to a particular field, whereas confirmation can easily be found for any theory which goes beyond finiteness [9].

The human mind, however, is not satisfied with these limits to the field of knowledge and therefore it continually reaches beyond what is knowable, thus entering the realm of *metaphysics*. Metaphysical concepts and theories share the following characteristics: they refer to totality, to the whole world, the universe or to other whole structures which cannot be made into an object of experience by a single scientist; they claim to be absolutely true, and they cannot be refuted.

Mechanistic materialism and holism are two examples of metaphysical theories; they seek in one principle the explanation of the whole of the universe.

In metaphysical theory, as we have seen, there is a tendency to convert an object which is present in thought (e.g. in holism the whole-making tendency) into an object existing in reality, i.e. to hypostatize it. Such conversion is evident with regard to the quest for the universal purpose. Hypostatization leads to the conclusion that God exists as the Designer of the universe, a proof derived from contemplating the purposeful arrangement which is evident in nature. Kant showed that his 'proof' of the existence of God is based on a fallacy. For it amounts to saying that, because we cannot *conceive* of nature save in the terms of the teleological idea, we are, therefore, justified in assuming the *existence* of a Being in which this idea is made absolute. (Kant, of course, realized that the existence of God cannot be disproved either, that religion is a matter of faith.)

Although God, as the absolute power responsible for the apparent purposefulness of scientific phenomena, cannot be accepted scientifically, the problem of the purpose which these phenomena exhibit has not been solved by denying the existence of the Designer. We shall confront it again in connection with the holistic, purposeful characteristics displayed by biological phenomena. What is evident is the necessity for eliminating the metaphysical aspect of absoluteness from the field of scientific knowledge, On the other hand, metaphysical thought itself, paradoxically, cannot be ignored in scientific endeavour.

Because of its anti-scientific tendencies, metaphysical speculation about the nature of things held up the progress of science for hundreds of years and this history, of course, still rankles in the minds of scientists who often identify metaphysical thought with philosophy as such. But metaphysical theories and concepts are not wholly inimical to science. In fact, they fulfil most essential purposes. The metaphysical impulse itself, the tendency of the mind to reach towards infinity, is a constant stimulus which never allows science to rest on its achievements. In this way, it is responsible for scientific progress.

Metaphysics is concerned with wholeness, which is, for the Kantian an idea, a guide to understanding. The whole is more than the component parts. To the metaphysician, the whole owes its form to a force which keeps it together, which is responsible for its organization. Thus, wholeness implies purpose (*telos*).

The section on holism showed the value of this idea for medicine. The living organism cannot be understood merely as an aggregate of parts. Smuts' teleological metaphysics was an attempt to account for phenomena such as the maintenance of body and mind in the face of external and internal influences, the phenomena of growth, regulation, adaptation, production of new wholes, and recovery from illness.

To the naive realist, the teleological principle exists as a power in nature; for the doctor, it exists in the patient. He relies on it as nature's power to heal as the resistance to disease, and as the ability of body and mind to adapt themselves to circumstances. This power acts as a *vis a fronte*; it pulls the child towards maturity, the patient towards better health.

When discussing holistic environmental treatments, we met a further manifestation of the teleological principle: the wholeness of society; the value of this treatment consisted in encouraging the individual person to integrate himself within the social whole.

Metaphysical thought does not only manifest itself in the hypostatization of the holistic concept; it also reveals itself in the structuring of scientific thought within the wholeness of a *system*.

The scientific system may be large or small, but whatever its size, the number of problems it entails is infinite; the search for knowledge goes on within its boundaries for ever.

A large system of which medical science forms a part is natural science. It includes biology and such systems as the study of the human body, of the individual organ and of the cell. Different organs serving the same function are united in such systems as the digestive, respiratory, nervous or locomotor systems, and cells compose a system represented by one particular organ. The concept of physical 'illness' or 'disease' leads to a further form of systematization. It acts as a framework which allows the doctor to assemble certain biological phenomena and thus make them comprehensible.

The mind stands for another system of reference. The individual man, however, cannot be fully accounted for by reference to his body or to his mind. He lives in a community with others. He belongs to a class of society. The social milieu is studied by sociology and this science in turn finds an application in social medicine, including social psychiatry. The community of which the individual forms a part, is affected by events which are studied by another science, moreover, namely history. Scientific thought, relevant to medicine, thus comprises aspects of natural science, of sociology and history. The principle of systematization in these sciences is derived from metaphysical thought. The idea of the system is evident also in the scientific *theory* which accounts for a class of phenomena. The inductive process of arriving at a general principle from the collection of individual observations ignores the fact that all these detailed phenomena are subsumed under the deductive theory which is a product of the creative mind and a further manifestation of the metaphysical urge.

Metaphysical thought thus provides science with constant stimulus for research, further knowledge being gained through forming *systems* appropriate for the particular phenomena. In these respects it is of great value to science. It also carries with it, however, the dangers of dogmatism and absoluteness. The doctor must be aware of these dangers. For example, a practitioner who uses the unspecific stimuli of natural therapy cannot absolutely rely on the holistic forces in the body, but must maintain, in readiness, those treatments which are based on the specific mechanistic-materialistic approach.

To the Kantian, the system is abstract, an organization of scientific thought, composed of concepts. It must be examined (epistemologically) regarding its nature, so that its scope and limitations can be ascertained. It is manifest in the scientific or metaphysical theory. To the naive realist, the system is part of nature and can be directly grasped by observation and experiment. Causality in the abstract system is an expression of *necessary* relationships, in the empirical system, causality is a part of nature, a 'cause'.

The doctor, working on the lines of the empirical naive-realistic approach, treats the patient's body and mind as natural systems; in physical illness he may find the cause of a painful swelling accompanied by a rise of pulse and temperature and by certain changes in the blood, in the presence of micro-organisms. If he accepts the epistemological Kantian approach, he is aware of the system of medical science, he realizes that he is interpreting the phenomena in his patient according to the sciences of bacteriology, immunology and pathology. In the case of duodenal ulcer two different ways of systematization, leading to different forms of treatment, were discussed in the Introduction, the two systems being mechanistic materialism and holism respectively. Both are metaphysical systems which lead to different scientific systems, to the use of different theories, concepts and treatments.

A special problem arises in the case of the psycho-somatic system. The two components are different in kind and the question of their relationship has been one of the most important and difficult problems in medicine and philosophy. This problem will now be discussed from the standpoint of naive realism and of Kantian epistemology.

THE RELATION OF BODY AND MIND

Emotional disturbances such as anxiety can cause physical changes, for instance in skin, bronchial tubes and blood vessels, and physical disturbances such as deafness or obesity can lead to emotional disabilities such as feelings of inferiority and depression. There is therefore no doubt that an interaction between body and mind occurs, but there remains the question of *how* this interaction occurs, from what general principle an explanation of the interaction can be derived.

Mechanistic materialism approaches the question of body-mind relationship from the angle of the body, explaining the relation itself in terms of particles and their forces: psychical life is understood as a function of the body. As was explained in the first chapter, it becomes a mere by-product of the brain in the philosophy of some behaviourists. Thus a monistic 'solution' of the problem of body-mind relationship is offered by mechanistic materialism: the mind is denied existence in its own right. This, we decided, is an unacceptable solution.

The holistic approach is based upon the activity of a hypothetical force in nature which tends to produce wholes. According to this view, body and mind merge as a unity in the human personality. This is certainly true, but the question of their relationship remains unanswered.

How does Kantian philosophy deal with the problem? It does so by effecting a fundamental change in the question itself. For it removes the two substances 'body' and 'mind' as two entities from the discussion, and thereby eliminates the search for the common denominator from which they are to be derived.

Kant approaches the subject from the standpoint of the 'Copernican Revolution'. It is no more a matter of two entities, body and mind, and their relatedness. It is a matter of *knowing* the body, the mind and the mode of their mutual relations as objects of knowledge. All knowledge is a manifestation of mental activity, the mind being the organ of knowledge. The mind occupies thus a central position, but, in addition, it also figures as one of the objects for knowledge, the body being the other object.

Whereas the naive realist assumes that any object can be known, the Kantian does not take the possibility of knowledge for granted, as he is aware of the limitations of knowledge. The principles which determine knowability have been stated. Applying them to the present problem, we arrive at the following position:

The body can be known, as it is finite and can be observed by a single observer. The mind, however, cannot be known; for it is infinite. Its lack of boundaries as a possible field for the scientist is connected with the fact that it has no extension in space, a point stressed by Kant [10]. As the mind is not an object of knowledge, the constitution of our cognitive faculty does not enable us to understand how these two fundamentally different phenomena, body and mind, are related. 'This is a question which no human being can possibly answer [11]'.

The application of Kantian epistemology to the problem of the relationship of body and mind thus leads to the conclusion that there is no solution for this problem, that in fact this is a pseudo-problem. It must, however, be emphasized that there is an essential difference between *empirical* detailed research into the interactions between bodies and minds and the epistemological question of the knowability of the common denominator and of the nature of the relationship. Scientists and doctors have to realize that the gap between the physical and the mental is unbridgeable. Whether we start from the bodily angle and follow nerve processes to the brain and across the 'gap' to the emotions or whether we begin with the emotions and follow their chain, say from an original emotional cause such as the fear of death to further fears of pain and suffering to the resulting emotional and across the 'gap' to the bodily conditions, the mode of the relationship between these states can never be known.

Philosophers and scientists who ignore the Kantian approach find themselves entangled in the mind-body problem. They do not realize the insolubility. Writers often make use of knowledge gained by neuro-anatomists 'which appears to constitute a bridge between body and mind; for emotions such as anger and rage can be localized in the brain, and the physiological basis of consciousness can be ascertained [12]. All these efforts at finding the bridge between body and mind fail; for the two realms are totally different, one has a spatial and a temporal extension, the other only a temporal extension. The mind is private, the brain is public.

If we follow A. J. Ayer and find a common denominator for body and mind in the human language, we are no nearer a solution to the problem; for, as R. Puccetti has pointed out, we have a dualistic language and we 'distinguish between our observations of events in somebody's body and our inference that he is having mental experiences of some kind [13]'.

As mental events are subjective, the neuro-anatomist who studies the connection between brain and mind would have to study the connection between his own brain and his own mind, *as his is the only mind he can know directly*; he would have to be equipped with mirrors in order to see his brain. Even if such experiments could be carried out, the results would not be applicable to other people, therefore they would have no objective scientific value [14].

The problem of the relation between man's body and mind cannot be solved by reducing man to the animal level. This course appeals to the scientists who imagine that in the animal they have a perfect model for the study of man. Such an approach is doubly misleading. For the question of relating an animal's emotion to its resulting physical state is no simpler than the corresponding question relating to human beings. One must assume that Pavlov's dogs, presented with juicy meat, had an *emotional* experience. It remains an answerable question how this emotional state is followed by the increased flow of saliva in them, even though neuro-physiologists can explain the action of the salivary gland or glands in terms of nerve supply.

The second mistake is concerned with the identification of man and animal. This is unjustifiable and leads to ignoring the ethical dimension of human life. It must be admitted that physical and chemical stimuli affecting the brain can have serious consequences for man's ethical judgement – the effect of alcohol is one example – and that mental illness, such as depression, also affects men's moral capacities; but in spite of these detailed empirical connections between body and spirit, and mind and spirit, it is wrong to deny man's spiritual dimension. (This question of medicine and ethics will be discussed fully in the next chapter.)

The fallacy of naive realism which accepts naively the physical structure of the brain as the basis for the mind, and the paradox which follows from this fallacy, have been clearly formulated by W. Riese as follows: 'Most contemporaries still cling, wittingly or not, to the *materialistic* thesis, according to which mental phenomena, abnormal or not, are the outcome of nervous structures and their activities. The adherence to this thesis stands in strange contrast to the inner world of *beliefs* and their manifestations displayed by physicians and scholars who, in matters scientific, would never yield to any metaphysic temptation, the materialistic thesis indeed being no more than an unrecognized and unidentified metaphysic raising matter to the power of *engendering* function, life and thought. Thus emerges the perilous dissociation of the modern scientist having two different thoughts, one for his laboratory and his research, the other for his interhuman relations, his attitude towards life and death, health and disease, his concept of man's place on earth and in the universe. As shown in a previous study [15], self-consciousness is the critical point at which the brain materialistic thesis collapses. The doctrine of concomitance breaks down at the same point. *Man simply cannot make his own self perceptible through any material structure whatever. Nor can any material structure serve as an intelligible "concomitant" of his self.* Were we to conceive both psychic and physical states as two states of consciousness or methods of *thought,* at least, the two things would no longer be "utterly differently" or incommensurable. The precise nature of their interrelation will still remain beyond human intelligence [16]'. . . . 'No anatomic investigation will ever answer the question of the interrelation of structural changes and mental behavior. It still seems to be as intelligible to us as to Aristotle and Galen to consider the structural changes as structural *conditions* of mental disease or, in more general terms, to conceive the brain, affected or not by lesions, as *instrumental* in mental behavior. Behavior may be changed by changing instrumental conditions, but not necessarily. This is but a restatement of our ignorance of the interrelation of mind and matter [17]'.

CONCEPTS AND PHYSICAL REALITY

When investigating the relationship between body and mind, we saw how Kantian epistemology could clarify the nature of the theories and concepts which scientists employ, thus resolving some of the difficulties into which naive realism leads them. We shall now apply the Kantian theory to the relations which obtain between certain concepts and reality in physics.

An important exponent of naive realism in physics was P. W. Bridgman. The divergence between him and the Kantian is seen at once in their respective attitudes toward the problem of the knowability of the world as such. According to Bridgman, 'the world we want to describe is in the first place the world of direct sensation [18]'. Description to him means knowledge, as is evident from the following:

'What our senses give us changes with time. . . . As we wait or move about or manipulate, we find certain correlations between the reports of our different senses, or between the reports of the same sense at different times. The establishment of such correlations is the first thing we do in getting order and understandability into our world. The thesis that there are such correlations is perhaps the broadest "scientific" thesis that we can formulate [19]'.

To this the Kantian replies that 'direct sensation' is unable to provide us with 'understandability' of the world, because it would amount to knowing the world as such, which is in fact unknowable.

According to Bridgman, physicists carry out operations which reveal aspects of the world. The operations are carried out with instruments such as microscopes or telescopes which are extensions of our eyes. 'Not only do we use instruments to give us fineness of detail inaccessible to direct sense perception, but we also use them to extend qualitatively the range of our senses into regions where our senses no longer operate, as when we detect and measure radiation phenomena at wave lengths beyond the sensitivity of our eyes, or acoustical phenomena above the range of our hearing [20] '.

To this the Kantian answer is that instruments and senses do not provide us with knowledge of the world, although they enable us to perceive the world. They aid the mind to test a theory which is abstract and composed of concepts which are, of course, also abstract.

According to Kant, empirical concepts derive from pure concepts ("categories of the understanding"). It cannot be denied, of course, that empirical concepts such as "energy" and "mass" find their application in reality; that they are applied to structures which are interpreted in the light of the particular theory (which is then checked through experiments and altered if the empirical evidence does not bear it out). But the theory itself is abstract and not part of reality.

It is thus significant that Bridgman is forced to admit that 'mass', 'momentum', 'energy' do not occur in the naked world around us. It is even more revealing that he should try to rescue 'empirical reality' by claiming that they occur only in conjunction with a nervous system and with activity in that nervous system of unfathomed complexity [21]. But, as the Kantian is quick to note, 'mass', 'momentum' and 'energy' do not arise from a nervous system – from the brain, a concrete structure, but are concepts which arise in the mind, in the abstract organ of knowledge. They reflect not 'the way things are' (the title of Bridgman's book), but the way the mind conceives the world.

The reader is already familiar with the Kantian approach to the problem of the relation between body and mind. The confusion into which the naive realist, who uses the mental (mind, consciousness) as interchangeable with the physical (brain) is led, is evident in the following statement by Bridgman: 'The knowledge that I have been talking about is the knowledge of ordinary experience as I see it in consciousness. If we ever become sufficient masters of the microscopic physiology of brain functioning to describe in full detail what happens during mental activity[,] it may well be that the activity which we call "knowing" may prove to have a strong component of probability in the sense that states of knowing which appear to conscious introspection to be the same[,] may have a microscopic structure varying over a wide range fixed by probability considerations [22]'.

In other words, knowing, an abstract matter, is considered to have a concrete spatial structure! This fallacious theory of knowledge leads Bridgman to the conclusion that the total amount of knowledge which can possibly be accumulated in the history of mankind in all branches of science is limited to the number of human brain units concerned with knowledge. Each unit can be instrumental in providing only a certain amount of knowledge. Bridgman is himself aware of this result, and he is left with the observation that 'the situation is highly unsatisfactory; it is even difficult to talk about it self-consistently [23]'. Thus the theory of naive realism breaks down in this particular case, having to admit inconsistency.

Another problem which arises in modern science concerns the nature of the electron. Here, too, the naive realistic approach leads to confusion. The difficulty is that the electron behaves in some experiments like a material particle and in others like a non-material wave. Therefore, it can be neither particle nor wave. The solution adopted by physicists in practise is to treat the problem mathematically, but the nature of the electron is still discussed.

The physicist A. Landé has taken a naive realistic approach to the problem, objecting to the idea that 'an electron is neither particle nor wave [24]'. He further denies that 'both particles and waves are mental pictures of equal rank [25]'. His argument is couched in classical terms and runs as follows: 'My answer is similar to that of the good Dr. Johnson rejecting the subjectivistic idealism of Bishop Berkeley: you can kick, and be hurt by, a stone as well as by a particle and by a water and electromagnetic wave; but you cannot kick, or be hurt by, a list of statistical fractions [26]'. In other words, knowledge, couched in abstract, mathematical, conceptual language, is here confused with a concrete, observable object. Such a mistake arises from the application of a naive realistic view.

The Kantian theory, affirming the abstract nature of knowledge, has no difficulty in accounting for the electron in a dual way. There is simply no contradiction in the fact that the physicist accounts for the electron by the use of two concepts, wave and particle. The late Sir James Jeans applied the Kantian viewpoint to the problem and explained the observed discrepancy in electronic behaviour by assuming that it was due to different kinds of knowledge and not to differences in the objects of nature. 'If the waves of a free electron . . . represent human knowledge, what happens to the waves when there is no human knowledge to represent? For we must suppose that electrons were in existence while there was no human consciousness to observe them, and that there are free electrons in Sirius where there are no physicists to observe them. The simple but surprising answer would seem to be that, when there is no human knowledge there are no waves, we must always remember that the waves are not a part of nature, but of our efforts to understand nature [27]'.

THE RELATIONSHIP OF MECHANISTIC MATERIALISM AND HOLISM AND THE SIGNIFICANCE OF THE TWO PRINCIPLES IN BIOLOGY

Our enquiry moves on from physical to biological reality, from dead to living things. We have reached the stage when we can gain clarity of the relationship of the two main approaches, mechanistic materialism and holism, in biology and of the significance of the two principles in this science.

Mechanistic materialism and holism lead to the two complementary approaches which are the means of studying living organisms: the former yielding knowledge of efficient causes through the isolation of parts and the latter arriving at final causes through relating detailed knowledge to the whole organism. Wholeness implies purposefulness, manifest in organized activity, the discovery and elucidation of which was defined by J. S. Haldane to be the task of biology [28].

As long as we maintain the naive realistic standpoint and take parts and wholes as knowable entities, we cannot arrive at an understanding of the character of the two complementary approaches nor can we discover the significance of the two principles in biology. We must change our orientation and go through the 'Copernican Revolution'. We are then concerned not with objects found in nature but with our knowledge of such objects; for reality as such is unknowable and particular phenomena, such as the constituents of nature, we realized, can be known only in the form of mental constructs.

Before we can determine the relationship between mechanistic materialism and holism, we must examine them separately from an epistemological point of view.

The knowledge which is the fruit of the mechanistic-materialistic approach represents all the detailed discoveries of biological science. Such knowledge refers to objects given in nature (although not knowable as such). When using this approach, the scientist *determines* his object of study with its aid, for instance the human body as consisting of a number of different organs, each being composed of a variety of cells. Mechanistic materialism provides thus the basis for the cognition of these natural phenomena; it is objective and constitutes scientific knowledge. Mechanistic-materialistic concepts are therefore *constitutive* concepts.

The holistic approach and the fruits which are the results of its application are entirely different in character. The principle of organization, of integration, this purposeful feature of the living organism, is not an element which enriches our knowledge of the objects further; its function is that it makes the results of research, carried out on mechanistic-materialistic lines, intelligible. We *reflect* upon the material which research has yielded and ask ourselves what function each part, for instance the heart or the kidneys, plays in the organization of the whole organism, in other words what the purpose of these parts is. Without such reflection, we cannot understand biological phenomena: our cognitive faculties require the teleological judgement. *Nothing in nature, however, corresponds to what we call the purposeful character, the organization, the integration of the parts.* Therefore the teleological judgement is purely *regulative*.

In fact, there is no purpose at all in natural phenomena. The notion of purpose is quite foreign to the objective realm of science; it represents a *subjective* element which scientists introduce into their work. Purpose, Kant reminds us in *The Critique of Teleological Judgement* [29], is an attribute of the human mind which is evident in intelligible purposeful thinking and in the actions which follow from it: 'We do not *observe* the ends of nature as designed. We only *read* this conception *into* the facts as a guide to judgement in its reflection upon the products of nature. Hence these ends are not given to us by the Object [30]'.

The teleological principle is used in biology 'on an analogy with our own casuality [31]'. An analogy, Kant points out, does not explain a phenomenon: 'Although this principle [of teleology] does not make the mode in which such products originate any more comprehensible, yet it is a heuristic principle for the investigation of the particular laws of nature [32]'. This last sentence entails an important assertion: nature in its teleological feature of life is inscrutable, and by comparing biological phenomena with our own purposefulness, by using the analogy with our own motivation, we do not arrive at an understanding of purposefulness. The scientist who has assimilated the Kantian viewpoints accepts this limitation with regard to knowledge; the naive realist, however, seeks vainly to eliminate the subjective character of the teleological principle and is led into confusion by his failure to distinguish between constitutive or determinant and regulative judgements and by making purposefulness into something objective. The difference between biological phenomena and physical structures can clarify the nature of biological knowledge [33].

Karl Jaspers has elucidated the dissimilarity between the natural and the artificial products from the point of view of scientific knowledge.

He has pointed out that the machine presents the investigator with only a limited number of problems and that these can be completely solved, whereas the living organism presents an infinite number of problems which can never find a final solution, but which always leave room for further research. The reason for this difference lies of course in the fact that one may can fully understand what another man has designed, that the machine has a designer, whereas the natural product is understood *as if* it had been designed [34].

Having gained insight into the nature of the analogical thought and of the mechanistic and teleological approaches as representing a constitutive and a regulative judgement respectively, the relationship between these two standpoints can be clearly seen. The position has been well summarized by J. C. Meredith in an introductory essay to Kant's *Critique of Teleological Judgement*: 'Owing to the nature of our understanding we are committed to the inadequate mechanical point of view to explain *how*, i.e. by what means, the end is realized in time, and so all we can do is to resort to the teleological point of view as a corrective. Both the mechanical and the teleological points of view are subjective, but their errors or inadequacies are of opposite tendency. So, by playing off the errors of one against the other we may hope to render the lens of human understanding achromatic [35]'. The two approaches are, however, not on the same level. The reflection as to the purpose of individual phenomena does not only come as an afterthought, as was indicated earlier, but the idea of purpose is a guide for the scientist throughout his work and 'we may regard the whole consistent *nexus effectivus* as subordinated to a *nexus finalis* [36]'.

The mechanical and the teleological points of view are subjective in so far as they both arise from the subjective human mental constitution. The mechanical approach is, however, objective so far as the validity of his results is concerned, whereas the teleological standpoint is subjective in the sense that it does not refer to anything objective in nature. Only by being aware of the character of these points of view can a scientist understand the implications of his own work. The naive realist is led astray by the shortcomings of his theory of knowledge. The significance of the 'Copernican Revolution' for biology can be demonstrated by an epistemological examination of the use of the teleological concept in J. Z. Young's writings which are concerned with the brain.

TELEOLOGY IN YOUNG'S CONCEPTION OF THE BRAIN

Young's conception of the brain was criticized in the first chapter. Objections were raised against his accounts of the brain as a calculating machine and against his recommendation of an engineering language for the description of cerebral processes. This physicalistic approach leads, for instance, to the identification of the memory of living cells and of minds with filing cabinets and to a physical interpretation of the information received by parts of the body and conveyed to others, in the shape of communication channels.

The choice of the physicalistic doctrine arises from a determination to avoid the teleological explanation of living phenomena, which are replaced by machines that function in accordance with physical laws. The naive-realistic standpoint in this treatment of living structures is obvious, as the scientist assumes that he can gain knowledge by observation of natural events as such and that such knowledge consists of an understanding of the mechanisms which are involved in the changes within the isolated parts.

To the Kantian, an event as such is unknowable, only a phenomenon or an appearance (i.e. what appears to the knowing mind) is knowable and is known by means of the mind's conceptual endowment. We saw that the mind uses the mechanistic-materialistic approach in constituting this knowledge. Young's theory of the way in which cells in the octopus' brain respond to visual stimuli is an example of such a scientific cognition of a particular natural phenomenon [37]: the shape of these cells is taken as the code which explains the mechanism by which the brain selects its reply from the available memory of stored representation. Apart from being a model for a mechanistic theory, the code, considered on its own, is a holistic device which embodies the idea of purpose. The brain's response to visual stimuli is an example of biological, purposeful activity.

The purposeful character of natural events is, however, unknowable, it cannot be grasped, but can be indirectly accounted for by a comparison with *human purpose*. The model of a machine is the obvious choice for such a reference, as the machine reflects the purposeful design of the mind of its inventor. Thus the regulative (as-if) character of the judgement of biological teleological phenomena is safeguarded.

When, however, a biologist like Young omits the inverted commas and reduces brains to homeostats or computers, he commits the error which consists in ignoring the difference between the regulative and the constitutive employment of teleology. This confusion leads to such absurd statements as the following: 'We learn [from machines] a language much more useful than the present one for speaking about brains and their "products" such as "mind" [38]'. As if the inert object which owes its origin to the thinking power of a living mind could teach a scientist's mind a language in which it expresses its own machine-thoughts and as if this 'language' could be of great use to the scientist in the understanding of his brain and of his own mind!

The 'Copernican Revolution' puts the matter right: the scientist's mind moves into the centre: it makes use of the teleological principle to account for cerebral phenomena. It coins theories and concepts which express this principle, such as those concerned with the biological aspects of memory. The teleological principle which is involved in these phenomena cannot be known. Certain parts of the brain are known *as if* they acted in a purposeful, memory-conveying manner.

The epistemological enquiry will now move on to the field of psychology.

NOTES

[1] See, for instance, A. J. Ayer, *The Problem of Knowledge*, 1956, Pelican Books, third chapter.

[2] See H. J. Paton, *Kant's Metaphysic of Experience*, Allen and Unwin, Ltd., 1936, 1st vol., p. 75.

[3] Immanuel Kant's *Critique of Pure Reason*, translated by Norman Kemp Smith, Macmillan & Co., London, 1929, p. 59.

[4] Sir James Jeans, *Physics and Philosophy*, Cambridge University Press, 1942, p. 144.

[5] ibid.

[6] ibid, p. 151.

[7] ibid.

[8] ibid, p. 152.

[9] See K. R. Popper, *Conjectures and Refutations*, London, 1963, Routledge & Kegan Paul Ltd., p. 36.

[10] See *Critique of Pure Reason*, transl. by Norman Kemp Smith, Macmillan & Co. Ltd., London, 1929, p. 353.

[11] ibid, p. 359.

[12] See for instance: A. E. Fessard, 'Mechanisms of Nervous Integration and Conscious Experience' in *Brain Mechanisms and Consciousness, A Symposium*, editor J. F. Delafresnaye, C. C. Thomas, Springfield, Illinois, U.S.A., 1954.

[13] 'Science, Analysis, and The Problem of Mind', *Philosophy*, 1964, vol. 39, no. 149, p. 254.

[14] ibid, pp. 252, 253.

[15] W. Riese and E. C. Hoff, 'A History of the Doctrine of Cerebral Localization, Pt. 1. Sources, Anticipations and Basic Reasoning', *J. Hist. Med. and Allied Sc.*, 1, 50-71, 1950.

[16] Chapter 4, 'The Neuropsychologic Phase in the History of Psychiatric Thought', from *Historic Derivations of Modern Psychiatry*, edited by Iago Galdston, 1967, McGraw-Hill, p. 104.

[17] ibid, p. 120.

[18] *The Way Things Are*, Harvard University Press, Cambridge, Massachusetts, 1959, p. 45.

[19] ibid.

[20] ibid, p. 149.

[21] ibid, p. 154.

[22]. ibid, p. 176.

[23] P. W. Bridgman, 'The Nature of Physical "Knowledge" ', contribution to *The Nature of Physical Knowledge*, ed. by L. W. Friedrich, Oliver & Boyd, Edinburgh and London, 1961, p. 23.

[24] 'Dualistic Pictures and Unitary Reality in Quantum Theory', contribution to *The Nature of Physical Knowledge*, ed. by L. W. Friedrich, Oliver & Boyd, Edinburgh and London, 1961, p. 88.

[25] ibid.

[26] ibid.

[27] *Physics and Philosophy*, Cambridge University Press, 1942, p. 171.

[28] *The Sciences and Philosophy*, Hodder and Stoughton Ltd., 1929, p. 84.

[29] Transl. by James Creed Meredith, Oxford, Clarendon Press, 1928.

[30] ibid, p. 53.

[31] ibid, p. 34.

[32] ibid, p. 68.

[33] Recent research, aimed at producing living structures from inanimate material, cannot affect the conception of life as distinct from physical matter. Even if it were possible to synthetize all the characteristic elements of the living organism, the living forms thus produced would take on the fundamentally new features and would show the characteristics of life with its own inscrutable teleology. The judgement of the organism is not influenced by the way in which it originates.

[34] *Psychologie der Weltanschauungen*, 2nd ed. Springer-Verlag, Berlin, 1922, p. 472.

[35] Kant's *Critique of Teleological Judgement*, Oxford, Clarendon Press, 1928, p. xxvii.

[36] ibid.

[37] See his paper 'Memory Mechanisms of the Brain', *J. of Mental Science*, March 1962, no. 453, vol. 108, p. 122.

[38] *A Model of the Brain*, Oxford, The Clarendon Press, 1964, p. 6.

PART II

Kantian Epistemology and Psychological Medicine

THEORY IN PSYCHOLOGICAL MEDICINE

The 'Copernican Revolution in Thought' has enabled us to resolve antinomies which the naive realistic approach cannot resolve. In the field of biology, we found that the two principles, mechanistic materialism and holism can be reconciled, and teleology was shown to represent a necessary regulative principle in the interpretation of living structures. We now have to apply the 'Copernican Revolution' to the psychological field and have to face the particular situation in this area.

The enquiry into the relationship of body and mind has prepared the ground, as it has revealed the fact that the mind is not a scientific object, as it is infinite. It is therefore a metaphysical object. This conclusion is of great significance for the theory of mental phenomena. As Karl Jaspers has pointed out, the theories in medical psychology are fundamentally different from the theories in natural science. Psychological theories show a lack of verifiability and of falsifiability, and there are no counter-theories. Thus he called psychological theories 'deceptive speculations about presumed existence, they have taken forms analogous to the theories of natural sciences but for the most part lack any logically clear method [1]'.

In his *Psychologie der Weltanschauungen* [2], Jaspers applied Kantian epistemology to psychology and showed why psychology cannot be a science in the sense of a natural science. He quoted passages from Kant's *Critique of Pure Reason* [3] which deal with the psyche and which refer to views earlier expressed in this chapter.

When discussing the relationship between science and metaphysics, I pointed out that a metaphysical theory tended 'to convert an object which is present in thought into an object existing in reality, i.e. to hypostatize it [4]'.

Accepting Kant's view, Jaspers called the psyche (or the mind or the soul) an *idea*. It stands for the totality of a person's experience [5] and for 'a simple substance which persists with personal identity [6]'.

Under the guidance of this idea, 'we connect all the appearances, all the actions and receptivity of our mind [7]', but we 'never attain to a systematic unity of all appearances of inner sense [8]'.

We are led to think of 'a single fundamental power' from which we can derive 'the properties' [9] of the soul, but this trend of thought is illusory: 'The soul in itself could not be known through the assumed predicates ... for they constitute a mere idea which cannot be represented *in concreto* [10]'.

The fact that 'the whole of understandable connections is never given [11]' means that knowledge in a systematic form is impossible in psychology. We must therefore qualify the earlier statement that 'the mind stands for another system of reference [12]'. It stands for a system of reference in people's thoughts, they think of it as a frame of reference, it is an idea that has a regulative function, but the mind is not an object which can be known by means of a system, a viable scientific theory.

In the section on science and metaphysics, the idea was referred to as an expression of metaphysical thought. Ideas stimulate us to aim at wholeness or totality, but such aim can in fact not be realized. The correctness of this limitation of knowledge is borne out by the different schools of Medical Psychology. Their theories will now be examined from the point of view of Kantian epistemology. I shall start with the psychiatric application of behaviourism.

THE IDEA OF A COMPREHENSIVE BEHAVIOURAL SCIENCE

In the first chapter, behaviourism was rejected as a form of materialism which identifies the mind with its neural correlate and which conceives it to function atomistically, following the pattern of stimulus-response. Behaviourism is, however, not restricted to this narrow interpretation. Some behaviourists accept the existence of psychic phenomena, but they are concerned only with their objective, observable manifestations, i.e. with overt behaviour. In such behaviour they see reliable information and data for knowledge which the subjective experience does not appear to provide.

Behaviourists vary with regard to the strictness of their approach. A very wide approach was chosen by Roy R. Grinker, Sr. in his paper entitled 'The Sciences of Psychiatry: Field, Fences and Riders [13]'. Grinker's exposition illustrates the consequences which follow from an uncritical adoption of the idea of totality.

Grinker aims at establishing psychiatry as a behavioural science. In order to achieve this aim, he has to integrate all the sciences, 'involved in understanding human behaviol [14]'. His list comprises biological sciences, namely genetics, general biology, anatomy, physiology, biochemistry and pathology, all the social sciences and psychology. He thus combines bodily, psychic and social phenomena.

In order to attain an integration of all psychiatric knowledge, Grinker expects the Freudian psychologists (no other school of medical psychology is mentioned) to agree to 'a shift in conceptual thinking' and 'to learn how to think in terms of information and communication, without the use of energic or topological language [15]', i.e. to adopt a behaviouristic character. The common denominator of all the relevant sciences is found in 'transaction' which includes 'information and communication', 'transactions with other individuals, groups or things', 'some physiological internal transactions' and 'some derived from the past (memories and role repertories) [16]'.

Actions and transactions are conceived as observable in nature, within the body as movements of cell constituents, within the mind as recalled memories and within the social field as relations between people.

The discovery of actions and transactions in the different fields which Grinker wants to unite is not enough. For the realization of his idea of a comprehensive behavioural psychiatry, he investigates 'basic principles applicable to the analysis of all systems of inquiry', into the 'organization, structural and functional wholeness, its relation to its parts and its environment [17]'. He uses analogies as 'one method of relating systems of varying order of complexity [18]'. These analogies are extraordinarily vague: 'the symbol in the human societal system is analogous with the gene in the genetic system: psychologically, learning is analogous with physical growth. Homeostatic mechanisms and variability may be analogized as a similar process from cell to society; part-whole relationships are certainly capable of being viewed as analogous throughout all systems [19]'.

Grinker himself is not satisfied that analogizing is more than a 'preliminary' method, in fact he admits that 'it adds little to our knowledge of relationships among systems'. He thus investigates each system with regard to its 'basic principles' and discovers that 'each system has a structure which is composed of integrated parts within permeable boundaries insuring openness. It has extent in time and space. Its form is derived from its past, its present has relative stability, and it has future potentiality. In and of itself, an organizational system is a patterned process of action which has a purpose in the living economy, representing respectable teleology.

'Each system resists disintegration by realignments of gradients, partial sacrifice of structure and function or by hardening its boundaries to decrease permeability and openness. Finally, each system is in patterned transactional processes with all others which constitute its environment, to a degree dependent upon intersystemic closeness, significance for viability and for stress responses [20]'.

The last sentence reveals the fallacy of Grinker's approach which is the fallacy of naive realism. Each 'system' is a system of thought, a theoretical structure, as such it is not transacting with another system; anatomy is different from the social sciences; its structure is similar to the structure of physiology and pathology. No system has an environment, although the human body has its surroundings, but as a body it is not composed of anatomy, physiology, genetics, etc. but of parts which are not knowable as such, but only as objects of a science, namely of the science of anatomy, and their functioning is knowable by means of the science of physiology.

Medical science studies phenomena occurring in the body and in the mind. Certain medical phenomena are the concern of psychiatry. Some of these are also studied by the science of biology, others by genetics, by psychology and sociology. A comprehensive behavioural psychiatry is an idea which cannot be realized. The human psyche cannot be explained in terms of transactional processes. Such an account reflects the deterministic conception of man which was criticized in the first chapter as the hallmark of behaviourism. It leaves no room for purposive action of an individual, for his freedom.

THE IDEA OF A SOCIAL PSYCHIATRY

We found that Grinker included the social sciences within his Comprehensive Behavioural Psychiatry. We must now enquire how Kantian epistemology can account for mental health and mental disease from the social point of view. We shall have to apply the conception of the mind, defined as an idea, to the social-medical field and relate the epistemological enquiry to the naive realistic approach of social psychiatry which was chosen in the first chapter.

The Idea of the Social Challenge in Psychiatry

Social psychiatry was described in the first chapter as a form of holistic environmental treatment, based on the individual person's need to integrate within a community and on the community's readiness to accept the individual within its holistic structure. The idea of the psyche must be applied to the two components, to the individual social mind and to the collective social mind.

At the beginning of this section, I quoted Kant's definition of the psyche as the idea under the guidance of which 'we connect all the appearances, all the actions and receptivity of our mind [21]'. Social actions and phenomena are subsumed under the idea of the individual man conceived as a social being. This idea is related to the idea of a community which affects the individual in a reciprocal manner.

By connecting phenomena within 'our mind', Kant approaches the psyche from a subjective, experiential point of view. We can adopt this approach and are led to the individual's experience of the community and to the community's experience of the individual. The relationship is ambivalent, and the pathological features of the relationship represent the negative aspect of the ambivalence, whereas social therapy relies on its positive side.

Man feels threatened by society, his individuality is endangered by their expectations, demands and values. Society feels threatened by the individual who is not prepared to conform to it. Thus the individual experiences society as a challenge and may be felt by society as a challenge to its own individuality.

A challenge involves a demand for action, it entails an acknowledgement of freedom. The pathology of social relations is the failure of the meeting of this challenge.

Emotional disturbances from early childhood onwards can be understood under the guidance of this idea. The child's integration within its family and the family's integration of the child, the challenge of the school, of a work community, of a social stratum, of a country – all these situations present social problems which individuals and their social surroundings have to attempt to solve.

The situation is aggravated when the individual is not wanted by the social unit. The pathology of the illegitimate child is an example of this kind. Although the adopted child is told that its adoptive parents have wanted it, it becomes suspicious, as it has been rejected by its natural mother, and it may feel that it owes gratitude to its adoptive parents. The person who has been forced to emigrate feels rejected by the country he has left and is not sure of the welcome by the next community. Any change of social surroundings causes a sense of insecurity which is liable to produce psychiatric symptoms.

Once a child or an adult has broken down mentally, the social unit in which he lives is under great strain through this member's mental condition, and the patient may become very sensitive to his social environment. Community Psychiatry tries to cope with the problem of the mentally disturbed patient by accepting the responsibility of providing the therapeutic environment. The psychiatrists, working in a community psychiatric hospital, must understand each patient's challenge and social problem as well as the social unit's problems.

The idea of the social challenge can guide the psychiatrist to collect material which is relevant for the understanding of the challenge in a particular case for the estimation of its force and for the resolution of the conflict.

Epidemiological Psychiatric Knowledge

There is room for factual studies within the framework of the idea of the social mind. Psychiatrists count sufferers from a particular mental or psycho-somatic illness within certain communities and publish these figures. This is a form of objective knowledge. We learn, for instance, from Berthold Grünfeld and Christen Salvesen that patients suffering from depressive, paranoid and hysterical psychoses tend to belong to a low social stratum [22], from R. E. and K. E. Gordon that young married women, particularly at the childbearing period, tend to break down emotionally in a 'rapidly growing suburban community [23]', and from J. Ph. Hes that immigrants coming to Israel from Oriental countries, tend to exhibit more hypochondriacal symptoms than those who have emigrated from Occidental countries [24]. All these studies give over-all pictures of mental illnesses in certain social settings. Such investigations suffer from the vagueness of such terms as 'hysterical psychosis', 'hypochondrias' and 'emotional illness' as well as from the vagueness of a definition of social strata and of specific cultures. No such study leads to the formulation of a law which could predict from what illness a particular person, living in a particular social environment, will break down. These studies are statistical calculations which point to the dependency of man on his various social surroundings.

Scientists aim at the formulation of laws which express invariant behaviour. As E. Nagel has pointed out, 'the fact that social processes vary with their institutional settings, and that the specific uniformities found to hold in one culture are not pervasive in all societies, does not preclude the possibility that these specific uniformities are specializations of relational structures invariant for all cultures [25]'.

The idea of social relations conceived as a challenge is the invariant from which the different relations and their vicissitudes can be derived.

The idea does not, however, imply that the social psychiatrist can predict what kind of moral challenge will be faced by an individual and by his social group.

The results of an epidemiological enquiry must be explained under the guidance of the idea of the social challenge. The patients who were included in the three quoted statistical surveys broke down under such challenges: the young married women could not stand the isolation in a 'rapidly growing suburban community', especially as looking after their young children presented them with another challenge; the immigrants to Israel found the challenge of the new country too much for them, and the people from the 'low social stratum' suffered from the handicap of their social position which presented them with a challenge which aggravated their psychotic conditions and proved an additional handicap which those coming from a better social class did not suffer.

The Fallacy of the Deterministic-Scientific Approach to Social Life

Social psychiatry as a science has no room for the moral factor of a challenge, but the challenge is an essential element in this field, as J. Leff, a social psychiatrist, has found 'evidence for the importance of family relationships in determining the outcome of psychiatric disorders'. To anybody who is aware of the important bonds between the members of a family, such finding simply confirms what is obvious. If the members of the family show love and tolerance toward each other, the sick person benefits. If, on the other hand, there is disunity, the patient suffers.

We learn from the same author that 'scientific studies of social intervention pose knotty methodological problems' and further that 'these have to be solved if social psychiatrists are to advance beyond interesting speculations to the identification of social causes of psychological symptoms'. [26] Such advance cannot be expected as the crucial factor of the moral challenge cannot be accommodated within the deterministic scientific framework.

The fallacy of deriving individual social phenomena from a deterministic theory becomes evident when such phenomena are compared with physical phenomena which can be predicted according to laws which are based on the presupposition of determinism.

E. Nagel has denied that determinism is less valid for the social phenomena than for physical phenomena and he has chosen two cases, taken from these two fields, to illustrate his thesis. In both cases, prediction failed.

The case, taken from the physical realm, is fictitious. He assumed that an anti-aircraft gun, equipped with a mechanism which calculates the direction toward the target, failed to hit the target because the signals which transmitted the calculations disturbed the adjusting mechanism.

The case, taken from the social realm, is a historical event: 'On the basis of an apparently adequate analysis of the state of American economy, economists predicted a business "recession" for 1947. However, because of this warning, businessmen lowered the prices of a number of products occupying strategic positions in the operations of the economic market, so that effective demands for the goods was increased and the predicted recession did not take place [27]'.

In the first case, the phenomena are in principle predictable in terms of the science which derives them from mechanistic determinism. In the second case, the phenomena are in principle unpredictable as they are the outcome of human actions and not of deterministic laws. People have a duty to prevent a slump in their own interest and in the interest of others, and in the case quoted they acted in the appropriate manner, manifesting human freedom. Where man fails to do his duty, he is guilty of irresponsibility.

Limitations of the Freedom of Social Actions

Man is not entirely free, although he is basically free and is not a robot, as we saw when we discussed the claims of mechanistic materialism. He is free to the extent to which he is in control of his actions which, in turn, stem from his conscious intentions. To the extent to which he is driven by unconscious motives, he is not responsible for his activities.

Social phenomena reveal man's lack of freedom. The individual may project unconsciously his own aggressiveness into his fellow human beings. In such a case he gets suspicious and cannot meet them as a responsible social partner. He may also unconsciously identify himself with a person who has had a great influence on him in his formative years (like his father) and who had anti-social feelings, expressed in anti-social actions. He may be full of resentment against the world, hating others as he hates himself. The seeds of such emotions, also leading to anti-social behaviour, may be buried in his unconscious mind.

A social group is easily swayed by irrational feelings of which the members are hardly aware. Mob violence due to panic is an example of irresponsible group behaviour.

Psychiatric social phenomena, such as the behaviour of psychopaths, illustrate the results of unconscious resentment. The attitude of society towards the mental patient illustrates the unconsciously harboured fears.

Apart from the social-psychological factors, social actions are determined by the individual's genetic endowment. Abnormal chromosomes have been found in delinquents.

Racial factors play a part in alcoholism. Jews show a low prevalence of this condition, whereas the American negro is very prone to it.

The individual can exercise his freedom in spite of the determining factors. As E. H. Erikson has pointed out, man strives unconsciously for achieving and sustaining a personal character, for an 'inner solidarity [28]'. He thus experiences the tendencies of identifying with others as a challenge and can resist such tendencies. The group can help the psychopath to overcome his anti-social disposition, as community psychiatry has proved, and can assist the alcoholic to keep off drink, as the record of Alcoholics Anonymous demonstrates. These examples confirm that man is fundamentally and potentially free in spite of the limitations of his freedom. The deterministic-scientific approach must therefore be subordinated under the idea of the ethical approach which is expressed in the notion of the challenge to which the individual and his group must try to find an answer.

The Idea of a Social Evolution

Man's faith in his freedom and therefore in himself is corrupted by scientists who abuse their authority and apply the naturalistic-scientific approach to social relations. Such an exposition offends against Martin Buber's correct appreciation of the 'between' in human relations. As he said, 'what is peculiarly characteristic of the human world is above all that something takes place between one being and another the like of which can be found nowhere in nature [29]'.

It has become fashionable to understand the 'naked ape' in terms of other animals. Sociologists study the social lives of insects, such as bees and ants, and of mammals such as deer and monkeys, and apply the fruits of such investigation to man. Culture, the expression of human values, becomes an evolutionary requirement. Konrad Lorenz in his book *On Aggression* gives many examples of such confusion [30]. He has equated culture with instinctual patterns which individual animals have to adopt. There is thus no moral challenge. He has expressed this naturalistic point of view as follows: 'The urge to become a member of a group, for instance, is certainly something that has been programmed in the pre-human phylogeny of man, but the distinctive properties of any group which make it coherent and exclusive are norms of behaviour ritualized in cultural development [31]'.

It may well be true that human beings require rituals and customs for their social life and that they have inherited some of their social habits from their evolutionary ancestors and share them with animals, but the nature of the challenge is totally different in the human being and 'the moral law within us' has *not* 'arisen by natural selection, just like the laws of heavens', as Lorenz maintains. To expect Kant to agree to such confusion, as Lorenz does, reveals a complete lack of understanding of Kantian philosophy [32]. As A. C. Broad has pointed out, 'unless the notion of value is surreptitiously imported into the definition of "evolution", knowledge of the facts and laws of evolution is simply knowledge of the de facto nature and order of sequence of successive phases in various lines of development [33]'.

The Idea of Social Psychobiology

The surreptitious introduction of the moral principle into an alleged deterministic-scientific social investigation is not confined to the study of the social evolution of the human race. The same fallacy is evident in the writings of those who derive interpersonal relations from the biological development of the individual person.

Harry Stack Sullivan's *The Interpersonal Theory of Psychiatry* [34] is based on the 'developmental approach' in which he sets out to formulate 'how, from birth onwards, a very capable animal becomes a person . . . and how this transformation . . . is brought about, step by step, from very early in life, through the influence of other people, and solely for the purpose of living with other people in some sort of social organization [35]'.

As a psychiatrist, Sullivan was particularly interested in the meaning and significance of anxiety, and he postulated that anxiety in a mother is transferred to her child.

While anxiety is often conveyed from one person to another, and especially from a mother to her child, the biological development of the child does not provide an explanation of this phenomenon. An example, taken from Sullivan's book, illustrates the fallacy of his approach.

Sullivan describes how a baby depends on his mother for being kept clean and says: 'the anal zone of interaction [between mother and child] thus necessarily comes to involve factors of an interpersonal character from very early life. The functional activity centering in the anal zone often becomes involved in the manifestations of infantile anxiety, especially when the [mother] is made anxious by these details of her mothering function. By this I refer to those who find it extremely difficult to deal with the infant's soiled diapers, and so on [36]'.

This account of the pathology of human interaction is at fault. The biological bowel function and the anatomical zone are not the root of the trouble, which lies in the fact that the mother cannot cope with the experience of handling her child's excreta without feeling anxious. Such a squeamish woman has to face the challenge of the situation. If she fails, she may well make the child anxious and spoil her relationship with the child and, perhaps, the child's future relations with other people. Thus an interpersonal relationship is a moral and not a biologically determined issue.

Teleology in Social Psychiatry

As an isolated person cannot develop his personality, the social situation fulfils a necessary purpose in human life. The pathology of social relations, however, expresses the individual's and his group's failure to meet the challenge.

The ethical approach which judges relations in society involves for a psychiatrist the consideration of health, an assessment of the situation as it *is* and not as it *ought* to be, a *deterministic* and not an *ethical* assessment. The idea of the social challenge has thus to be subordinated under the idea of *health* which is a teleological idea that requires clarification.

Health stands for wholeness in the single body, the single mind and in the social unit, whether it is a family, a community in a village, town or country. As in the case of the body, we judge the individual or the collective mind under the guidance of the teleological principle.

The healthy body and the healthy mind differ fundamentally from the epistemological point of view. The difference lies in the fact that the body is an object for science and the mind is not. The body is composed of parts which are studied in isolation, it is known scientifically by means of their relationship to each other, i.e. their mechanisms. Although we can distinguish special functions of the mind, cognition, sensation and volition which are investigated medically (as are the bodily functions) and studied by psychiatrists in their various abnormal conditions, the mind is not 'known through the assumed predicates' as Kant taught us. As we are concerned with the social predicates, we apply the idea of the mind to them.

The person whose cognitive, emotional or conative capacity is disturbed may not be able to make the social relationship expected of him. He is socially sick, in need of social therapy.

The Kantian definition deals with the individual mind and not with the collective mind. It is essential to examine them separately from the teleological point of view.

The relationship between two individual minds is fundamentally different from the relationship between individual bodily organs or functions, such as respiration, circulation and assimilation. The latter serve the whole of bodily maintenance for its harmony, whereas it is a feature of the interhuman relation that it involves tension, the challenge being the expression of this feature. A healthy interhuman relationship is one in which the two persons confirm each other in their uniqueness and tolerate each other in their differences.

The teleological notion of the collective social mind has been criticized by E. Nagel. He has shown that for such an explanation to be valid it would be essential to specify the state of the system and the variables which are related to each other and which are required to maintain the system as a whole [37]. Following Nagel's argument, we must admit that social units are far from stable (as bodies are stable) and that the individual social mind is often related (or ought to be related) to fluctuating groups which split up. It is true that there may be a certain distinctive spirit in a certain family, a class of children, a hospital community, etc.; the spirit is not necessarily permanent and groups may disperse without dying in the sense in which a living organism dies. The medical point of view does, however, assess such units as whole structures and as health-promoting or health-endangering to the individual on account of features such as tolerance, enthusiasm or hatred and anger. The medical judgement of social relations is thus different from the moral judgement. The latter stresses unselfishness, whereas the former stresses the stamina which are required in such relationships and traces the mental breakdown to the imbalance between the person's stamina and the demands made upon them. Social mental health is thus a teleological idea in which the ethical social demands are recognized and are subordinated under the medical requirements. Social therapy follows from this conception, it aims at strengthening the social capacity of the individual and the readiness of his social group to meet him in his social endeavour.

If social psychiatry is not conceived under the guidance of the teleological medico-ethical principle, but is conceived as a system comprising different components which are on the same level, confusion results. An example of such a mistaken conception is Norman G.

Hawkins' *Medical Sociology, Theory, Scope and Method* [38]. In common with other authors, Hawkins constantly switches from sociological to psychological and biological concepts. He thus arrives at such formulations as 'personal reorganization may be physiological, cognitive, and affective, or cultural [39]'. These diverse aspects of the human being are then incorporated teleologically into one 'system', as the sentence which follows the one just quoted shows: 'In any case, because the system reorganizes as a system and not as parts, the line of action will be influenced by considerations with reference to culture [40]'. There is no 'system' which comprises physiological, cognitive, affective and cultural reorganization.

Hawkins recognizes the need for distinguishing man from the animal. He thus postulates that 'man is an open system constituting a teleological, non-animal matrix [41]'. The concept of the 'matrix' is used to formulate an 'interdisciplinary outlook', to 'deal' with the 'the social, emotional, and cultural elements in health and sickness', to 'focus' attention upon 'break-down, pathology, and recovery as a single process, thus preserving the unity of the field' and to 'provide' through 'the principle of continuity of group and individual, organism and environment ... a common ground for epidemiology and ecology, social etiology, and the analysis of health service organization [42]'.

The fruits of this unified enquiry are a mass of unsupported statements such as that gastric ulcer, rheumatism, allergies, arthritis, and high blood pressure are due to stress and represent the manifestations of the emotional crisis of cultural, environmental stress, and the startling assertion that 'there is no essential distinction among the various stresses resulting from overwork, worry, poisonous fumes, germs, or economic insecurity, except that the type of disease which may eventuate is strongly influenced by whichever predominates at that particular point where malfunctioning makes necessary a decisive change in the "frozen function" known as organic structure [43]'.

For a correct interpretation of the cited phenomena it is necessary to differentiate between bodily and mental health. 'Poisonous fumes' are certainly unhealthy and so is 'economic insecurity', but their effects are quite different. Scientific knowledge is not furthered by Hawkins' universal teleological approach. Scientific knowledge is furthered by the discoveries of mechanisms involved in health and disease. With regard to physical health, the scientist has to find out *how* poisonous fumes (which may have something to do with a social situation, such as working conditions) affect a person's health. With regard to psychosomatic conditions, structural lesions result from the relations between the mind and the body, as I discussed earlier on. Tension, recognized by

Hawkins as the source of imbalance, exists in body and mind, but bodily tension is different from mental tension, as the body is different from the mind. The teleological principle must be applied in different ways to the physiological and the psychological effects of tension. The bodily organs are understood as if they were acting together purposefully, hence tension must be conceived in terms of this regulative use of teleology, as if it interfered with the purposeful collaboration between the different organs. The 'worry' and the 'economic insecurity' which constitute mental tension, on the other hand, must be conceived as a direct challenge to the person's conscious and unconscious purpose to meet his obligations, including those which arise from a social conflict. To state that the mental tension is causing the breakdown is a platitude. To discover *how* a particular person experiences the tension is the therapeutic task. This subjective approach, combined with the ethical approach, will be discussed in the next chapter.

THE IDEA OF THE INDIVIDUAL PSYCHE
IN MEDICAL PSYCHOLOGIES

The *Therapeutic Community* represents an application of teleology to social psychiatry. It has been pioneered by M. Jones. He conceived this community as 'the product of a union between psychiatry and the social disciplines' and he stressed the contributions from 'the disciplines of sociology and anthropology, of epidemiology and ecology, and of preventive and therapeutic medicine'.

The emphasis is on patients' behaviour: disturbed behaviour is controlled through the social interactions of patients and staff, through a sharing of responsibility. 'The daily examination of social interaction and difficulties . . . means that the patients become aware of many of the factors which lie behind behaviour and learn a great deal about each other's problems.' [44]

What lies behind behaviour is the way in which people experience their lives and what controls abnormal, antisocial behaviour and the acceptance of responsibility is their conscience. This moral factor is crucial for the telos, the achievement of social 'normal' behaviour. This factor cannot be integrated within the various sciences, quoted by Jones in support of his approach.

The individual acknowledges the challenge of his life in relation to his conscience, but he does not only think of his obligations. He also thinks of himself, his psyche, as 'a simple substance which persists with personal identity', as Kant said [45]. This 'substance' is an idea, as we saw. It provides the means of orientation for the subjective experiences of a person and for the objective connections. The schools of medical psychology investigate the psyche as a subject of science. They make the individual psyche an example of the genus psyche, as the individual body is an example of the genus body. Such treatment denies the uniqueness of the individual person which is expressed in the meeting of his challenge. As it views the psyche as an object of science and not as an idea, it rests on false epistemological premises. We shall now examine the consequences which arise from the scientific approach of the three main schools of medical psychology, the Freudians, Adlerians and Jungians. Kantian philosophy will again be used as a guide.

Kant admits that 'it is quite permissible to *think* [of the psyche] as simple, in order, in conformity with this *idea,* to employ as the principle of our interpretation of its inner appearances a complete and necessary unity of all its faculties', but he warns us that 'this unity can never be apprehended *in concreto* [46]'.

Naive realists do not heed Kant's warning. They are not aware of the limitations of knowledge, as their minds are focused on objects and not on the nature of knowledge of these objects. They thus ignore the difference between the idea and the object of knowledge. Freud, Adler and Jung were naive realists and their followers have repeated the fundamental epistemological mistake. I shall now examine the consequences which follow from their mistaken epistemology.

Freudian Psychology

An epistemological examination of Freudian psychology can distinguish between three underlying principles: (a) the hermeneutic; (b) the naturalistic-biological; and (c) the historical principle. These elements are interlinked in Freudian thought, but require separate discussion.

(a) THE HERMENEUTIC PRINCIPLE

Psychological medicine is concerned with man's fantasy life, with the numerous symptoms of emotional illness, with anxiety and delusions, with compulsive thoughts and actions and with moods of depression and of elation, etc. Many of these phenomena are part of so-called normal life as well. What do they mean? The answer to such a question can be given if a form of symbolism is accepted as fundamental, and the symbolism becomes the clue for the interpretation of the particular phenomena.

Wilhelm Dilthey, deeply impressed by the importance of Kantian epistemology and convinced that the philosopher must investigate the presuppositions of all types of phenomena, developed the idea of a science of interpretation, a theory of the principles of understanding and interpretation, a hermeneutic. In his essay *Die Entstehung der Hermeneutik* [47], he defined this approach as follows: 'We mean by understanding the process in which from signs given to the senses we come to know a psychic reality whose manifestations they are [48]'.

The 'signs' which the medical psychologist receives are not received by his senses, the patient receives them in his own subjective experience and conveys them to his therapist who interprets them in the light of his particular hermeneutics as symbols.

The critical therapist is aware of the particular hermeneutic which he has chosen for the interpretation of psychic reality. Freud was uncritical and refused to admit that his hermeneutic, sexuality, might not be universally valid. When Jung suggested to him that the sexual aetiology of neurotic illness might be valid only for certain cases, he replied: 'I feel a fundamental aversion towards your suggestion that my conclusions are correct, but only for certain cases (points of view instead of conclusions). That is not very well possible. Entirely or not at all. . . . There is only our kind or else nothing is known. . . . So now I have confessed all my fanaticism [49]'.

The important fallacy in Freud's reply to Jung does not only lie in the generalization of the sexual aetiology of mental illness, but in his unawareness of the very nature of his reasoning: it is not a 'conclusion' drawn from observations, it is not 'knowledge' of human nature (which as such is unknowable). The sexual instinct is made into the leading concept of a theory, and patients' symptoms and dreams are interpreted in the light of this theory, as if there was empirical evidence, a cause-effect relationship, where there is, in fact, a symbolic, hermeneutic form of reasoning, a point of view.

Having 'established' the 'truth' of man's sexual nature, the 'facts' of biological needs of instinctual gratification and striving for pleasure of gratification follow as consequences.

There is no empirical test for this hermeneutic but there is the evidence of sexual disturbances, of malfunctioning of the sexual instinct in many neurotic patients and there is the enormous response to Freudian thought in our age and the coming into the open of sexuality from its hidden position to which a former age had forced it.

In Freud's system, the symbol is fitted into a theory which claims the status of science. As Ernst Cassirer has pointed out, such a theory 'becomes a Procrustean bed on which the empirical facts are stretched to fit a preconceived pattern [50]'. He held that 'the principle of symbolism, with its universality, validity, and general applicability, is the magic word, the Open Sesamé giving access to the specifically human world, to the world of culture [51]'. As Karl Jaspers has said, 'symbols are infinite, accessible to infinite interpretation and inexhaustible, but they are never reality itself as an object which we could know and possess [52]'. A symbolic grasp of the world is thus magic and equivocal, whereas a scientific grasp is rational and unequivocal.

(b) THE NATURALISTIC–BIOLOGICAL PRINCIPLE

Freud's biological hermeneutic forms the basis for his naturalistic framework, for the naive-realistic standpoint according to which the psyche can be understood and treated as an object of natural science [53]. In the first chapter, the system of psycho-analysis was described. It was found to be modelled after a machine, a control apparatus, the ego taking the part of the controlling force and the material which it controls being mainly the instinctual energy (apart from the stimuli arising from the environment). The ego and the id are conceived in layers, and the deeper layers of the ego and the whole of the id lie in the area of the unconscious. In this scheme, the unconscious becomes the cause of the conscious, thus a man's feelings and decisions are not his own, but are the result of his unconscious. The therapist faces the patient with the 'truth' of the unconscious which is thus made conscious, and which is taken to be the 'cause' of his disturbance. He is not faced with *one* of the 'causes', allowing for a different non-instinctual aetiology.

While Freud's interpretation of the sexual instinct can be at least partly accepted, his interpretation of *aggression* must be rejected completely. In his theory, aggressiveness becomes a primary, fundamental human attribute, 'an innate, independent instinctual disposition', 'the most powerful obstacle to culture', 'the derivative of the death instinct [54]', held in check by the cultural super-ego.

Freud was led to the postulation of the death instinct by his clinical observations of sadistic and masochistic phenomena and of depressive illness. The concept thus appears to be empirically justified. In fact, aggressiveness is misrepresented empirically.

Karl Mannheim, a sociologist, found that man's peaceful and aggressive or warlike attitude depended on the particular social *milieu*. In *Man and Society* [55] Mannheim said: 'Since the innate psychological equipment of men leaves equally open the possibility of their becoming either warlike or peaceful, it depends on the nature of social institutions and of social régimes, whether man in the mass has a character of one kind or the other [56]'. Mannheim found that 'generally it is the food-gatherers and the agriculturalists who are known to be peaceful. Furthermore, trade and commerce very often make for peace [57]', but he admitted that 'it is dangerous to generalize, for under certain conditions the same factors might foster war [58]'. Thus the social conditions and not the fundamental instinct determine man's aggressiveness [59].

People's aggressiveness is not only brought out by a social situation, but also by a treatment situation in which they are expected to prove their therapists' views. Patients are highly sensitive to the analyst's expectations. The general public who read Freud's books or hear about them are less vulnerable, as they can preserve their critical faculty better than the patients, but they also are liable to suffer from the general pessimistic conception of the primary destructive urge.

Not all Freudians accept the metaphysical concept of the death instinct, but many accept the dynamics according to which 'we have to be aggressive to save ourselves from self-destruction ... This is true of neurotic aggression, which always operates destructively against the self within when damned up by anxiety and guilt and [when] it is so blocked from outward expression [60]'. This theory is naturalistic-realistic, as it postulates the psyche as a knowable part of nature and aggression as one of the fundamental elements within the psyche.

Aggressiveness is a subjective feeling and its power in so-called normal and in neurotic people cannot be denied. The medical psychologist who sets out to translate the subjective realm into an objective field of enquiry and who chooses the biological concept of instinct for objectification cannot do justice to this emotion; for it becomes an absolute power within the totality of experience which to him is the psyche, whereas, as Jaspers, following Kant, has pointed out, the psyche is in fact not knowable although we refer all experiences, including aggressive feelings, to the psyche as to an idea in our minds.

In the neo-Freudian literature to which I referred in the first chapter, aggressiveness plays a prominent part. According to Melanie Klein, the baby feels aggressive towards the mother's breast, towards the mother as a whole and towards the father. W. R. D. Fairbairn developed the neo-Freudian theory and conceived the libido as 'primarily object-seeking (rather than pleasure-seeking) [61]'. Fairbairn was convinced that psycho-analysis reveals man's true measure of aggressiveness associated with his sexual tendencies [62] and developed a complicated theory of the manifestation of the repressed aggression.

Fairbairn traced aggressiveness to hatred which is said to be a prominent force in the early oral phase of instinctual development:

'The great problem which confronts the individual in the early oral phase is how to love the object without destroying it by hate ... Any disturbance immediately calls into operation the hating element in his ambivalent attitude; and, when his hate becomes directed towards the internalized object, a depressive reaction supervenes [63]'.

As some Freudians do not accept the theory of the death instinct, there is also some disagreement with regard to the universal validity of the theory of aggressive object relations. O. Fenichel, for instance, held that there 'is certainly no reason for assuming that every infant sucking at his mother's breast has the desire to kill and destroy her in a sadistic manner [64]'.

From the point of view of Kantian epistemology, the criticism must not only be directed against the generalization from the findings of certain analyses to all breast-fed children and in fact also to those who were not breast-fed (which is Fenichel's criticism), but, more fundamentally, against the assumption that one attribute of the psyche determines human nature absolutely — human nature being unknowable.

Therapists and their patients observe emotions empirically, they also, as I said before, evoke them because the theory demands their existence, but they do not observe empirically the significance of the libidinal object relationship. This significance follows from the Freudian or neo-Freudian theory which is not derived from the observed phenomena, as empiricists hold, but from which, on the contrary, the significance of the phenomena is derived. The theory itself, as a theory of the constitution of the psyche, is irrefutable and metaphysical, and is not scientific.

The objective theoretical approach leads to the conceptualization of feelings which are concerned with values: people feel guilty and bad when they experience their own hatred and aggressiveness. But, as Fenichel has emphasized, 'a scientific psychology is absolutely free of moral valuation. For it, there is no good or evil, no moral or immoral, and no what ought to be at all, for a scientific psychology, good and evil, moral and immoral, and what ought to be are products of human minds and have to be investigated as such [65]'.

To the scientist, the value-free investigation of phenomena is indeed the only concern, but to the human being, feelings of guilt have a moral value and the genuineness of this value must be respected.

The subjective and the moral quality of emotional life which is revealed in aggressiveness cannot be dealt with within a naturalistic-biological framework, such as the Freudian. It can be accommodated in a framework which is based on subjective experience and which allows for conscience, i.e. for freedom, the opposite to scientific determinism. Such a basis for the understanding of patients will be discussed in the next chapter. The findings of Freudian naturalistic-biological psychology will then have to be re-interpreted.

(c) THE HISTORICAL PRINCIPLE

The Freudian naive realist is not only unaware of the true significance of the theory which he has adopted and of his method of hermeneutics, but he is also oblivious of the significance of the historical principle. All these principles lead him to the assertion of absolute determinism, expressed in the presupposition of causality, the hallmark of science.

The historical element is intimately connected with the symbolic and naturalistic-biological interpretations. The Freudian man is the product of the libido which moves him through its manifestations and phases; his emotional state at any one time is explained as the result of a previous state. Not only is the present taken as determined by the past, the past is interpreted in the light of memories and of material dug up from the unconscious relating to the past. Human nature, fixed in the hermeneutic, undergoes in the naturalistic-biological scheme changes without being able to change its nature. During the analysis, the patient's ego is subjected to experiences which gradually cause it to 'give up' its 'defences' and 'resistances' which the therapist 'unmasks' in the chronological order of the sexual development. Thus there is no personal freedom, only historical-libidinal determinism.

The deterministic picture is at fault; for the patient must choose to submit to the treatment and must be willing to face its painful aspects; also he must want to get rid of his illness. Thus the therapist relies on his patient's freedom to decide and to cope with his life. It is only within the 'scientific' framework that there is no freedom.

History, conceived as a chain of cause and effect, becomes man's fate, whereas history, conceived as a moment of decision and of encounter, becomes man's freedom. The individual patient asserts his freedom in the therapeutic situation; confronted by his unconscious feelings and motives, his sexual and other urges and his need to change. The freedom of this historical decision will be further discussed in the next chapter; it is connected with the subjective, non-scientific approach.

To the Kantian, there is no conflict between historical causality and personal freedom. For he has recognized the fact that causality is not in the phenomena but in the mind of the scientist who presupposes it so that scientific knowledge can be attained.

Historical knowledge is different from the knowledge of natural science, as it is the knowledge of the individual and not of a class. This individual aspect of history plays a part in the Freudian treatment. A sexual trauma, for instance, is interpreted as a personal historical event and the state of the patient is explained as its result. The trauma is thus not related to an impersonal ego.

Historical time must be differentiated from physical and biological time. As E. P. Papanoutsos has pointed out [66], 'we often make the mistake of imagining historical time after the manner of Euclidean space, which is homogeneous throughout all its extent ... but the time (historical, as I prefer to call it rather than psychological) in which human life is played out is not thus neutral [67]'.

From a subjective point of view, historical time is experienced in a meaningful manner, from the objective scientific-historical point of view it is punctuated by events which the historian must take into consideration in his historical researches, i.e. in his understanding of the historical period which he studies. These events, as Papanoutsos showed, include personal decisions. They are not the only historical causes which explain the final historical events or the historical development; biological and sociological causes must also be taken into consideration. In addition, psychological causes are operative, and their power has been revealed by Freud and his followers as largely operative in the unconscious; for people are moved by unconscious motives, they may identify themselves with a father or mother without being aware of such cause of their action. If the person becomes aware of these influences he has the possibility of making his decision, thus asserting his freedom.

The historian judges the character whom he is studying from a moral point of view and considers him to be responsible for the consequences of his actions and may find him guilty. The individual person, whether a patient or not, judges himself from the same point of view. The chain of historical causality does not in any way rule out such judgement. Psychotherapy increases the individual's freedom as it diminishes the power of the unconscious by revealing it to consciousness.

In the historical moments of analytic therapy the patient faces himself, his past and present, and thus actualizes his freedom. This situation is in no way contradicted by the factors which determine man, physically, biologically, or sociologically. The Freudian who follows a naive-realistic and naturalistic-biological approach is caught in the determinism of his 'science' and considers man's freedom an illusion. Such a view corrupts man. The remedy lies in the awareness of the foundations of knowledge, which is the Kantian endeavour.

Adlerian Psychology

Freud's naturalistic scientific approach was bound to fail, as the psyche is not an object of naturalistic science. The hermeneutic-naturalistic-historical determinism conveys to the people who accept the Freudian view the idea that they are the victims of fate, an idea which is harmful to them.

Alfred Adler, who broke away from Freud, claimed to have established a true science of the mind and to have avoided the mistakes which he discovered in the Freudian system. He expressed his faith in man's freedom and denied the efficient causality which makes psychoanalysis deterministic. I shall now examine the Adlerian approach from the standpoint of Kantian epistemology.

The outstanding concept in Adler's psychology is *teleology,* and the examination of this concept on Kantian lines can clarify Adler's Individual Psychology. Teleology was used ambiguously by Adler. We shall now discuss two meanings in which the term is employed in Adlerian writings.

(a) Teleology was to Adler an attribute of nature; as such it stood for an objective *metaphysical* power. H. L. Ansbacher and R. R. Ansbacher refer to this type of teleology in their book *The Individual Psychology of Alfred Adler* [68] as follows: 'The science of Individual Psychology developed out of the effort to understand that mysterious creative power of life which expresses itself in the desire to develop, to strive, and even to compensate for defects in one direction by striving for success in another. This power is teleological, it expresses itself in the striving after a goal, and, in this striving, every bodily and psychological movement is made to cooperate [69]'. This teleology is holistic. It was described in the first chapter as an absolute principle, in Smuts' words: 'the motive force behind evolution [70]'. To the patient, the therapist's belief in a creative, whole-making power may well be inspiring, but confusion sets in if the therapist claims that he makes this concept the cornerstone of his science; for, as we learnt from Kant, wholeness is an idea under which the scientist can subsume phenomena, but it is not a scientific concept.

The holistic view is manifest in Adler's acceptance of the principle of homeostasis which he saw expressed in the interaction between the different parts of the body: 'Organs are related to one another as though in a secret alliance, along with the gland of internal secretion . . . and they are able to give one another reciprocal support [71] '. As Smuts applied the teleological 'principle to account for more and more complex structures, so Adler applied the holistic conception not only to the body, but also to the psycho-somatic whole: the inferiority of the body was to him compensated for by strong mental development. He went still higher up in the scale: the most important whole which was decisive for his orientation as a psychotherapist and as an educator was 'the ideal society' which he called 'the ultimate fulfilment of evolution [72] '.

Neurotics, psychotics and delinquents were judged as having opposed 'the goal of perfection', 'the urge of evolution', they 'violate reality [73] '. They must suffer, as 'deviating to any extent from the truth must lead to the injury of the person . . . if not to his overthrow [74] '.

As we saw when discussing social evolution as an aspect of social psychiatry, the concept of this evolution is a hybrid which has been derived from naturalistic-deterministic Darwinism and from non-naturalistic ethics. The concept may act as an ideal for politically-minded people, but it cannot act as a guide for psychotherapists. The adoption of the concept does not only lead to bracketing neurotics with delinquents, but also to consider all emotionally sick people to be pampered and spoiled. As I shall show in the next chapter, such treatment can seriously prejudice the therapist against his patient. Thus evolutionary teleology cannot be accepted in psychological medicine.

(b) The second use of the notion of teleology is connected with the first. It, too, is supposed to form the scientific basis for Individual Psychology. The relationship of the first and second type of teleology can be clearly seen from the following sentences, quotations from Adler's writings: 'I found man to be a [self-consistent] unity. The foremost task of Individual Psychology is to prove this unity in each individual – in his thinking, feeling, acting, in his so-called conscious and unconscious, in every expression of his personality. This [self-consistent] unity we call the style of life of the individual [75] '. These 'expressions' of the 'style of life' are not only viewed as manifestations of the objective holistic teleology, but also as the *subjective* manifestations of the psyche.

According to Adler, the style of life is established in very early childhood. 'Everyone carried within himself an opinion of himself and the problems of life, a life line, and a law of movement which keeps fast hold of him without his understanding it or giving himself an account of it [76] '. This subjective opinion causes each individual to choose his subjective goal which determines for him his values and his meaning of life. The striving for this goal is taken as the clue to a person's life and to his neurosis.

In violation of the social interest, the neurotic is found to strive for superiority; he is driven to this goal by his feeling of inferiority. The self with its creative power is credited with the ability to change the subjective goal, hence Adler's psychology with its internal, subjective causality is not deterministic in an absolute, but only in a relative sense ('soft' determinism).

The emphasis on subjective experience is a most valuable part of Adlerian psychology. As I mentioned in the discussion of Freudian psychology, the subjective element will be discussed in the next chapter. The subjective approach does not, however, yield scientific knowledge which is objective and generally valid. As Adler stressed the uniqueness of every personality with its unique subjective striving, he could not generalize, although he claimed that he could often predict the movement of the life style in an individual person, but, he frankly admitted, he might be wrong in his prediction.

The subjective approach which is valid in psychotherapy (although not as a scientific approach) suffered serious confusion in Adler's writings as a result of his acquaintance with H. Vaihinger's 'Philosophy of the as-if'. In contradiction to Kant, Vaihinger denied that the mind of the scientist can build up knowledge which is objective and independent of the individual scientist's emotional life. To Vaihinger, scientific thought was fictitious, pragmatic; objective truth did not exist, a scientific object, logical principles and moral maxims – all were to him just useful fictions.

Adler's application of Vaihinger's philosophy caused him to interpret the life-style of his patients as fictitious in Vaihinger's sense. In fact, although the patient imagines the goal, within the framework of his subjective life, it is real – in Kantian terminology, the telos is constitutive and not regulative. We must understand him, not as if he had an aim, say of gaining superiority, but as somebody who in fact *has* this aim.

It is true that the wrong subjective aim precludes a person from adapting himself to objective circumstances but the objective circumstances do not represent reality in an epistemological sense, but in a psychological sense. The confusion of the Adlerian application of Vaihinger's philosophy can be seen from the account which Lewis Way gave of it in his book *Adler's Place in Psychology* [77] : 'The individual seems to live according to a fictional pattern which his scheme of apperception has imposed upon reality [78] '. To the Kantian, apperception of reality consists of perceiving phenomena in the framework of space and time and of raising them to the status of scientific knowledge by means of certain *a priori* concepts such as causality. The validity of this apperception was denied by Vaihinger. The apperception to which Adler referred is the appreciation of one's role in society, avoiding such mistakes as considering oneself superior or inferior to others. These wrong 'fictions' are corrected by the Adlerian therapist, whereas Vaihinger's 'fictions' cannot be corrected at all.

Adler's subjective approach is foreign to objective naturalistic science, but, Adlerians have argued, such science is not the only science. They have accepted Wilhelm Windelband's distinction of two forms of science, the 'nomothetic' kind which formulates generally valid laws – natural science being of this kind – and the 'idiographic' kind which discovers the laws pertaining to the individual. Adler's Individual Psychology has been classified as an example of 'idiographic' science, although his adherents have also claimed that the principles which he 'discovered' such as the striving for superiority, the social interest and compensation for organ defects are generally valid, 'nomothetic' principles.

I have already demonstrated that these principles are in fact not scientific, the term being used in the 'nomothetic' sense. It now remains to examine the 'idiographic' claim.

Alexander Neuer, one of Adler's pupils, investigated the scientific status of Individual Psychology and came to the conclusion that the Adlerian understands the individual scientifically from a subjective-teleological point of view 'idiographically', as the historian understands the individual person who is the object of his study [79]. In order to gain the essential objectivity, Neuer argued that the individual's subjective life is known in terms of the objective, teleological force which makes him strive upwards, and which expresses itself in the style of life and in such emotional qualities as courage, anger, lust for power. Neuer thus expressed the subjective teleology in terms of the objective teleology. But this form of teleology is, as we have seen, metaphysical, and therefore cannot serve as a unifying concept for a science of the individual psyche.

Jungian Psychology

Jungian psychology provides another example of the confusion which arises when a thinker is unaware of the dangers of naive realism. The whole psyche became an object for Jung's enquiry which he claimed to be scientific, whereas we saw that the psyche is an idea which is beyond the reach of scientific knowledge. Thus in spite of his commentator's J. Jacobi's insistence that Jung's 'statements always refer to empirically verified facts and are strictly limited to what is conceivable on the basis of experience [80]', Jungian statements are in fact metaphysical. They can be grouped under three headings, comprising an ontological, a dualistic and a holistic principle.

1. JUNGIAN ONTOLOGY

The term 'ontology' is meant in its metaphysical sense as the science of Being. Jung's psychology is ontological as he conceived the psyche to be 'set up in accord with the structure of the universe' and as he held that 'what happens in the macrocosm likewise happens in the infinitesimal and most subjective reaches of the psyche [81]'. Thus knowledge of the macrocosm and of the microcosm is claimed by him who presumes to know the common structure of the universe.

The individual person becomes determined in this ontological framework. His personal conscious and unconscious are based on a collective unconscious. 'The collective unconscious is common to all; it is the foundation of what the ancients called the "sympathy of all things" [82]'. Jungian ontology thus postulates the existence of a universal harmony. The common source from which humanity has originated is said to be endowed with organs through which it exercises its power: the archetypes. This ontological structure is reflected in different ways.

(a) Michael Fordham, one of Jung's prominent pupils, has elaborated the *biological* aspect of the archetypes [83]. He has quoted Jung's view that 'all the psychic processes accessible to our observation and experience are somehow bound to an organic substrate [84]'. The biological, archetypal theory identifies the archetypes as 'hereditary functions' and concludes that 'they must be somehow represented in the germ cells and that therefore any archetypal image recorded by the conscious mind likewise contains within it the effect of genetic factors [85]'. The biological substrate is also located in the instincts and 'the archetypal images are the representatives in consciousness of the instincts themselves [86]'. The biological theory relates archetypes to instincts, to endocrine glands and to the central nervous systems. Instinctual patterns are influenced by hormones, for instance in mating, and depend on neural patterns. The argument then proceeds to bridge over from neurophysiology to analytical Jungian psychology, the nervous system has a rhythm, so have music, dancing and sport, apart from other activities: Jung's 'research' has 'closed' the gap, interrelating these different 'manifestations [87]'.

(b) The biological, neural manifestation of archetypal ontology is linked with the sphere of *symbolic* imagery. The link is made through the 'discovery that the stimulated neurones in the brain form patterns on the cortex [88]'. Fordham, quoting Jung, accepts the idea that a symbol, now understood as 'inner', i.e. mental image, 'always pre-supposes that the chosen expression is the best possible description, or formula, of a relatively unknown fact [89]', postulating that the fact exists, presumably in an organic manner.

The symbol, made by the archetypes, is understood as proceeding from every psychic function. The symbol has a 'transcendental' function, binding together 'incompatible opposites of which man appears, not only psychically but also physically [90]', thus manifesting the universal harmony of the underlying ontology.

The symbol defies rational expression and explanation. It has an 'irrational component we can grasp only with our feelings [91]', it is a picture or image in the irrational realm of the unconscious and is experienced as meaning in the conscious sphere. In contrast to Freudian psychology, Jungian psychology sees in symbols living things which give rise to mystical experience, they 'give metaphysical reality to a cosmic system in which God is central, ultimate and incomprehensible [92]'.

The collective non-rational unconscious expresses itself symbolically in dreams, phantasies and hallucinations: apart from the archetype God, it produces the symbol of the feminine and masculine principle (anima and animus), of wisdom in male and female shape (wise old man and wise old woman) and others.

(c) The collective unconscious does not just provide man with symbolic experiences, it is also a *power*. Through its archetypes it controls man, and man is compelled to face the archetypal powers. Symbols are laden with energy, they control the 'undifferentiated and primitive libido [93]', and archetypal energy, Jungians warn us, can destroy the personality if it invades the conscious layer suddenly.

The power of the archetypes is seen by Jungians in bringing about phenomena of synchronicity, a coincidence of events which has meaning for the people concerned. Michael Fordham has given an example of such intervention by archetypes: A man was taking part in a boat race which his father had come to witness. He had been in conflict with his father. The archetypes took a hand: 'the mast fell overboard for no apparent reason, and put the boat out of the race [94]'.

2. JUNGIAN DUALISM

Jung and his followers have described the way in which the archetypal power works. The outstanding characteristic feature lies in its dualism. The dualistic principle is evident in the different spheres of archetypal activity: in the archetypal ruling of the individual person and of the universe.

According to Jungian thought, 'the self is the original archetype of infancy [95]', it is 'the real power behind the manifestations of our psychic life . . . the urge towards consciousness and wholeness [96]', its counterpart is the ego, the conscious side of the personality. The two assume different significance during the individual's life: in the first half, the ego is developed at the expense of the self, in the second half the self takes precedence. The symbols of the mandalas, the magic circles, are whole figures, but they are subdivided symmetrically, i.e. in a dualistic fashion. There is inner and outer life, life and death, consciousness and unconsciousness and the two types of extraverts and introverts.

3. JUNGIAN HOLISM

The opposite poles must be assimilated by consciousness, the psyche is conceived as a self-regulating system, the symbol of individuation describes the psychic wholeness. The 'psychological law' is harmony and integration: 'The end is always to bring a variety of colour, form, and aspects into a harmonious, organic unity, a "whole" [97]'. 'It is in the unconscious fantasies that the synthetic forces are to be found and when these forces become free, either in the course of normal growth or of successful therapy, dynamic changes occur within the individual which lead to a greater unification of his divided and conflicting parts [98]'. Where the individual fails to achieve adaptation and integration, the self has to regress to an earlier stage of development in order to achieve the missed holistic state. M. Jackson has applied the holistic conceptions which are valid for the body to the psyche which he understands and treats on the lines of Jungian psychology: 'If the physical organism has its maturational and defensive-repair processes, its compensatory reactions, its inflammations and immunological responses, why should it be so difficult to envisage the psyche as having similar functions or repair and growth? Just as the fever is not the infective process nor the repair process in itself, but is an overt sign of the activity of the underlying invasion-healing process, in the same way the neurosis can be regarded as not the healing process nor the pathological process itself, but as an overt sign of an underlying invasion-healing struggle [99] '.

EPISTEMOLOGICAL EVALUATION OF JUNGIAN PSYCHOLOGY

The last quotation, taken from Jackson's paper, reveals the naive-realistic character of the Jungian approach and the fallacies of the ontological-metaphysical underlying theory. Jackson argues naively: we have a body which functions holistically and we have a psyche which functions in the same manner. He assumes that body and mind are entities which are knowable as such and which are held together by holistic processes. In fact, the 'processes' to which Jackson refers are not as holistic activities part of the body, but are part of a science which uses teleological concepts and which considers bodily phenomena analogous to human intentions (as if they were purposeful). As the body can be observed objectively by a scientist, he can formulate a refutable theory composed of (abstract) concepts which he can apply to the bodily phenomena checking its accuracy.

The mind, however, cannot be observed objectively by a scientist, no scientific refutable theories can be devised, only metaphysical irrefutable statements can be made. These refer to human nature and to the universe as a whole. The 'forces' which Jungians 'discover' and which, they claim, represent the 'laws' of the psyche have nothing to do with scientific discoveries and scientific laws.

As the individual psyche is not an object of science, but an idea under which psychic phenomena are subsumed, theories which 'explain' psychic phenomena by reference to underlying 'strata' have no scientific validity either.

The connection of conscious activity with collective unconscious forces is open to the following objections:

1. The archetypes, arising from the collective unconscious, are supposed to be the 'a priori determining constituents of all experience [100]'. It is obvious that no science can deal with *all* experience, nor with 'a priori determining constituents' of experience, only with the causes or antecedent events of certain experiences.

2. The fateful power of the archetypes is absolute and thus reveals the non-scientific nature of the theory. The alleged symbolic character in which this power manifests itself raises a further issue which Karl Jaspers has stressed.

3. We can investigate myths, religions, dreams and delusions of patients and can thus obtain objective knowledge of symbols. Such

study does not, however, entail any belief in the power of the symbols which include God and sacred mandalas. Thus, 'psychological understanding of symbols moves among perilous *ambiguities* ... We get to know about them but only from without and our beliefs are not involved [101]'. The consequences of this ambiguity become clear when the 'knowledge' of the symbols is applied. 'We would like to heal through communicating our knowledge of symbols', Jaspers says, 'We want to bring them to life in ourselves, and invite participation in them [102]', but we suffer from a confusion, as knowledge and belief have different meanings which 'get inextricably mixed [103]'.

If we confine our attention to the facts of existing symbolic phenomena and do not consider the question of belief in them, i.e. if we deny them their power over us, we can follow Jung and discover parallelisms and even identities in different symbolic expressions of the human mind.

The discovery that the delusion of a patient treated in 1906 resembled the text of a Greek papyrus which was first edited in 1910 was to Jung of great importance and a proof of the existence of the collective unconscious which appeared to speak the symbolic language in mythological images to mankind eternally. The patient, a schizophrenic, had seen a solar penis, the papyrus speaks of the sun and a dangling tube. The patient had the delusion that he was God and Christ; the papyrus refers to the paths of the visible gods appearing through the sun, the God, my Father [104].

Jaspers has pointed out the flaw in this type of argument. The essential element is the *significance* of the symbol which is their effective content. It is very doubtful that the solar penis had the same meaning for the schizophrenic which it had for the writer of the Greek papyrus. The patient felt that he was God or Christ and he saw a penis dangling from the sun. Thus a genital element entered into his delusion, most likely the result of his personal sexual urge. The papyrus simply referred to God and to the sun and a dangling tube. Jaspers has put his objection to the Jungian theory as follows: 'Looking at these analogies more closely we find they are superficial and confined to general categories. For example, the point of similarity in dying and rising gods (Osiris is killed, Dionysius torn to pieces, Christ crucified) does not constitute their essential nature. The analogy throws light on what is inessential [105]'. If the symbols have in fact different meanings to different people, their therapeutic value cannot lie in their common language, arising from the common ground of the 'collective unconscious', as it is their *meaning* which constitutes the therapeutic factor.

Thus the study of comparative mythology and dream symbols becomes an exercise of historical-cultural, but not of psychotherapeutic significance.

4. While it is in order to compare different myths, dreams and manifestations of mental illness and while one can take such phenomena as manifestations of human phantasy (even if similar images may have dissimilar significance), the connection of the psychic archetypes with biological concepts is indefensible. Jung's view, quoted earlier, that 'all psychic processes accessible to our observation and experience are somehow bound to an organic substrate' was amplified by him in his paper *On Psychical Energy* [106]: the brain has been shaped and influenced by the remote experience of mankind, 'mental processes created physiological paths'. 'Impressive' experiences become bodily 'impressions'.

There is no justification for such views; neurologists have not discovered any shaping influence on the brain by any experience, and no path has been localized which can be said to have been made by archetypal experiences.

Michael Fordham's 'biological, hereditary theory', quoted earlier on, is another effort to bind the non-material archetype to the material germ cells. As we were informed, he found it necessary to assume that the 'hereditary functions must be represented in the germ cells' so that the 'archetypal image contains within it the effect of genetic factors'. We were told by Fordham that this feat must be achieved 'somehow', but not how.

We learnt further from the same author that archetypes are related to instincts which, in turn, are related to the endocrine and nervous system. 'Rhythm' is found to be the common denominator in all these activities. But is the rhythm of a dance and the rhythm of instinctual activities the same? The whole of this argument is conducted in the form of vague analogies and has no scientific validity. Fordham appears himself to sense the dilemma: he speaks of the localization of cerebral nuclei as arising from a mechanistic concept, and of the localization of the archetypal images as 'dynamic units' which function as whole and thus follow from a 'finalistic and purposive' approach [107].

EPISTEMOLOGICAL CONCLUSIONS REGARDING INDIVIDUAL MEDICAL PSYCHOLOGY

The epistemological evaluations of Jungian, Adlerian and Freudian psychology have confirmed the correctness of Kant's view that the psyche is not an object for scientific enquiry and that therefore scientific theories of psychic life cannot be formulated. Because the psyche is unsuitable for such treatment which is suitable for the body, all attempts directed at applying to the psyche the methods appropriate for the body are bound to fail [108].

We are therefore left with the science concerned with the events in the brain which affect the mind and with the science of genetics as it applies to mental health and mental illness. There is no doubt that further research will reveal more details of cerebral functions and their relations to individual mental conditions. Pharmacological discoveries will enable physicians to use drugs which have a profound effect on mental illness, and perhaps neuro-surgery will also contribute to the treatment of mental disease. Genetic studies may enable doctors to prevent mental abnormalities.

The organic approach in psychiatry has been linked with the psychological, but such scientific connection is not based on the psychological element, but on the organic aspect. An example is the relationship between responses to drugs and types of people. W. McDougall investigated the effect of alcohol on different types of persons and found that the extraverted person is more sensitive to this substance than the introvert [109]. Thus the Jungian typology is used in an objective, refutable investigation which enables the scientist to account for different biochemical responses. McDougall's theory does not, however, imply the acceptance of Jung's metaphysical theory according to which 'the extraverted attitude is characterized by an outward flowing of libido' and 'the introverted attitude' is defined, 'in contrast' as 'one of withdrawal', one in which 'the libido flows inward and is concentrated upon subjective factors, and the predominating influence is "inner necessity" [110]'. Nor does McDougall's employment of the Jungian typology imply any agreement with the Jungian view of a compensatory relationship between the two attitudes, one being conscious, the other unconscious. McDougall observed the relationship between the subjective attitude and objective pharmacological data.

While the Jungian concepts of introvert and extravert can be fitted into a scientific organic theory, his concept of archetypes, his central theoretical concept, cannot find a place in science. We saw that Fordham's attempt directed at the formulation of a biological theory of archetypes broke down. The alleged psycho-dynamics of analytical psychologies cannot be integrated within the dynamics of organic scientific psychiatry, for the latter accepts the critical standard of empirical science, whereas the former does not, but reigns supremely in a world of dogmatic, irrefutable absoluteness.

The theory of schizophrenia can serve as an example. The organic school seeks an explanation of this condition in physical abnormalities. C. E. Frohman and his co-workers claimed that they had discovered certain metabolic abnormalities in schizophrenic patients [111]. A. Mangoni and his collaborators checked this claim and did not confirm these findings [112].

In contrast to such refutable, tentative theories, the psycho-dynamics of Jung and Freud incorporate schizophrenia within their metaphysical systems: according to Jung, the disease is due to an 'intrusion into consciousness' of the archetypes of the anima and the animus which 'live in a world quite different from our own', and this 'intrusion' often blasts into fragments the all-too-feeble brainpans of unfortunate mortals [113]'. According to a Freudian, 'some schizophrenic symptoms are direct expressions of a regressive breakdown of the ego and an undoing of differentiations acquired through mental development (a primitivization). Other symptoms represent various attempts at restitution. The first category of symptoms embraces phenomena such as fantasies of world destruction, physical sensations, depersonalization, delusions of grandeur, archaic ways of thinking and speaking, hebephrenic and certain catatonic symptoms. The second category embraces hallucinations, delusions, most of the schizophrenic social and speech peculiarities, and other catatonic symptoms [114]'. The worlds of the Freudian ego and of the Jungian archetypes are thus not part of the world of science. They are metaphysical worlds, fashioned after the world of science.

PSYCHIC DETERMINISM AND FREEDOM

The Human Personality

There are laws of mental functioning which are discovered by empirical methods. In the first chapter, the laws of suggestion were mentioned. The mind of the person who is the target of another person's (or of a number of persons') suggestion acts in an almost automatic manner. His whole personality can be affected, his feelings, his attitudes, his values; his movements obey the suggestion, and many of his bodily functions are also influenced. Suggestion may be intentional or unintentional, may be beneficial to a person's health or harmful.

We learnt that Charles Baudouin explained the effects of suggestion by postulating that they affected the subconscious mind, giving rise to an idea which realized itself in the various phenomena.

Baudoin's theory has to be modified. The laws of suggestion are not valid for all minds, the suggestions are the more effective the more they meet a person's own wishes. Furthermore, they express a will and they impose themselves upon a will. Therefore behind the apparently mental object is a personality, a subject, who directs the functioning of the mind (and indirectly the body) in hetero- or in auto-suggestion.

What applies to the mechanisms which are set into motion by suggestion, also applies to such mechanisms as association of ideas which explain the sequence of thought-contents and to the Gestalt psychology which accounts for the structure of perceptions. None of the mental mechanisms, whether they are normal or abnormal, explain the functioning of the mind, although they are all referred to the mind, they are viewed under the idea of the mind. The body is explained with reference to its mechanisms, heart beat, blood circulation, respiratory movements, etc., all of which are viewed under the auspices of the regulative teleological principle. The comparison with the body clarifies the position of the mind.

The human personality gives distinction to a mind and gives relevance to the separate mechanisms. As Karl Jaspers has pointed out, 'personality is the term we give to the *individually differing and characteristic totality of meaningful connections in any one psychic life* [115].

Individuality entails freedom from elements which are foreign to it, whether it relates to feeling, to cognition or action.

Action is the outstanding feature of the personality, it must be distinguished from activity or movement. Charles Taylor has pointed out that action must be accounted for 'independently of its antecedent conditions or the laws by which it is explained [116]'. He has clarified the difference between action and movement as follows: 'To say that action is irreducible to movement is to say that the statement that an action has been done is never equivalent to the set of statements describing movements [117]'. Action is irreducible to movement, 'even if these statements characterize the movements in terms of the conditions they result in; for a movement which brought about a given result is still not the same thing as an action which was directed towards this result [118]'.

Taylor's example illustrates the vital difference between movements and actions: 'If I claim that someone tried to hit me, and adduce his movements as evidence, I am not generally talking about the movements which his limbs in fact underwent, but rather about his *directed* movements, i.e. his actions. I infer that these movements could have no other aim, given the circumstances, than striking me. If it is shown that the man was completely asleep, the *premiss* of the inference collapses [119]'. There is room for unconscious intention in Taylor's account: as he says, I may admit that I intend to seek justice by an action directed against someone, but I may in fact intend to avenge myself and may be unaware of my (unconscious) motive [120].

If I speak of behaviour in terms of movement and in terms of actions, I am guilty of ambiguity, as Taylor points out [121].

The neural explanation of mental phenomena is fallacious because of this ambiguity. There are movements in the nervous system, but there are actions of the person, the result of his (mental) decisions, desires and intentions. The bodily movements and their mechanisms cannot account for the mind. As we saw when discussing the relationship of body and mind, scientists in fact reserve for their own minds the non-deterministic, non-scientific approach even if they postulate a materialistic so-called scientific neural interpretation for the mind of their scientific objects.

We must distinguish between animal and human action. The animal and the human being both act purposefully, for instance when avoiding a painful situation, but only the human being, when his mind has achieved a certain state of maturity, acts with responsibility and appreciates values and meaning in a moral sense.

If psychologists ignore the significance of action and the difference between man and animal, and if they use a deterministic scientific framework for the understanding of the mind, they arrive at grotesque conclusions. They claim that they formulate personality theories, but they do not do justice either to the personality of an animal nor of a man. Of course, they observe what follows from their premise, from the presupposition that the mind and its environment form a system which is composed of units which act on each other in a necessary manner. Two examples from a collection of papers entitled *Current Perspectives in Social Psychology* [122] can illustrate the confusion which results from this approach.

J. McVicker Hunt set out to test a hypothesis according to which the organism interacts with its environment. The reaction of the organism is said to be determined by the information received from the environment, 'the input' and by its seeking of 'incongruity' which implies a striving for new situations. This outgoing effort is, however, limited so as to avoid too incongruous information. The 'proof' of this theory consists in the observation of college students, monkeys and rats. They all got bored if kept in a monotonous atmosphere, but they did not venture out too far and became fearful when confronted with 'dissonant information', 'when the inputs from a situation were too incongruous with the information already coded and stored [123]'.

The following objections must be raised against this theory:

1. Although it presumes to be a psychological theory and tries to account for mental states such as fear and boredom, it is in fact biological by nature, as it relates these states to the condition of the 'organism'.

2. In so far as the theory attempts to explain mental phenomena, it avoids a teleological explanation, reducing the mental phenomena to an atomistic level. As was pointed out earlier, Charles Taylor has shown that such a reduction is not possible [124].

3. The theory reduces human to animal action. It is true that people, monkeys and rats get frightened if they are confronted with too much 'incongruity', but the human being can be expected to stand up to such a situation, even if 'the inputs . . . are too incongruous with the information already coded and stored [125]'; in other words, man is expected to show courage which is not demanded of animals. Thus his actions alone are governed by the moral principle and his freedom is the freedom of responsibility, while both man and animal share the freedom of purposeful action.

Purpose entails motivation, and motivation is the central concern in another paper, entitled 'Motivation Reconsidered: the Concept of Competence'. The author is Robert W. White [126]. To White, the essential capacity of the organism is competence, which refers 'to an organism's capacity to interact effectively with its environment [127]'. Competence is said to have 'a motivational aspect', for this aspect we need some 'energy' which White discovers in the 'neuro-muscular system'. He quotes 'playful and exploratory behavior [128]' and admits that we cannot form a satisfactory idea of such phenomena on a neural basis. The aim of motivation is 'the satisfaction of effectance [129]' which is evidence from 'a feeling of efficacy'. The whole 'acquition of motives' is described as 'a complicated affair', 'yet', White suggests, 'the satisfaction of effectance contributes significantly to those feelings of interest which often sustain us so well in day-to-day actions, particularly when the things we are doing have continuing elements of novelty [130]'.

Motives are said to serve to produce 'realistic results in the way of income and career [131]'. The 'feeling of efficacy' thus depends on a judgement of the results of motivation. If a person is satisfied with the state of his income and of his career, if he finds himself sustained in his day-to-day actions, if he can meet new·situations, then he concludes that his motives have been correct. There is thus a reflection on values, and the feeling of 'satisfaction' which White relates to 'a trend of behavior [132]' is an indication of having adopted the right motives. White mentions the role played by 'unconscious fantasies of a sexual, aggressive, or omnipotent character [133]'. Such unconscious motives often cause feelings of guilt, i.e. dissatisfaction with one's motives, once they have reached consciousness or while the motives are judged by an unconscious conscience. Motives are thus judged from a moral point of view, and although we are moved by them often without being aware of their nature and force, we accept feelings of guilt, a feeling of dissatisfaction with ourselves, a reminder to investigate the nature of our motives. After we have become aware of our motives, we are free to change them if we consider them to be unworthy.

White does not accept such a theory which is based on the presupposition of freedom. His theory is founded on the presupposition of determinism. 'Effectance motivation' is 'neurogenic'. White's theory is nonsensical; for the cells of the nervous system cannot feel satisfaction nor dissatisfaction. Motives are of the mind and not of the body. The fact that our minds are motivated and that we feel satisfied or dissatisfied with our motives is further proof that the mind cannot be understood in scientific-deterministic terms.

Although the mind is not an object of scientific knowledge and mental phenomena cannot for this reason be fitted into a deterministic system and explained by a theory of the personality, we must assume that it is partly determined by its connection with the body and by its own inherent mechanisms, by its history and the social *milieu*. The bodily determining factors form part of the biological scientific system, the genetic factors form a system of their own which is expressed in symbolic language. The purely mental determinants such as mental illness (in distinction from brain illness), temperament, strength and weakness of personality are the factors which limit the freedom, the potentialities of an individual's mind. Their influence can be gauged by psychological and clinical-psychiatric tests, by intelligence and aptitude tests for instance. Thus clinical psychologists and psychiatrists can measure special functions and abilities of the mind and can assess a patient's progress by comparing the results of such measurement at different stages of the treatment. Thus objectivity of science is possible within the field of the mind. What is not possible is to formulate a theory from which laws of mental functioning can be derived. The question whether such laws exist is idle, as laws do not exist outside the realms of science, they are not 'in' the mind, as they are not 'in' the body, but owe their existence to the equipment of the scientist's mind [134].

THE EVALUATION OF HUMAN RELATIONS IN MEDICAL PSYCHOLOGY

The libertarian and the deterministic principles are thus both valid in medical psychology. This contradiction is only apparent, as a reconciliation of these principles is possible. The patient is considered primarily as a free person, but his freedom is taken to be limited by the determining factors. Medical judgement assesses his freedom and his determinism.

The deterministic aspects of the patient's personality can be formulated in a lawful, statistical manner; the libertarian aspects must not be so formulated, but the patient's freedom must be expressed in terms of his individuality in relation to other individual persons and his responsibility towards them and towards himself. Freedom must take precedence over determinism. An example can illustrate the situation.

D. Bardon and his co-workers treated women whose mental illness had arisen during pregnancy or within twelve months of their confinement. They treated the mothers with their babies in a mental hospital [135]. The libertarian aspect of such therapy is based on the assumption that each mother feels responsible for her baby, and for the relationship which the child needs for its emotional growth and which the mother needs for her own emotional development.

The authors of the paper recognized this postulate, as they said: 'an essential part of the treatment regimen was the encouragement of the mother to assume complete responsibility for the care of the infant as quickly as possible [136]'. The authors also recognized the responsibility of the staff in relation to the mothers' freedom: 'it was necessary for them [the nurses] to check their own strong maternal feelings and at the same time to encourage the mothers to care for and handle their babies [137]'.

Each mother's ability to carry out her maternal responsibilities has to be assessed as a measure of her individual freedom. Because of the mental illness, there was a risk of infanticide and of lack of interest in the child. The mental illness itself was treated on scientific-deterministic lines: anti-depressant and tranquillizing drugs as well as electro-convulsions were employed.

Although these physical measures are obviously essential, they are secondary to the psychological treatment, the making of personal relationships between the staff and the patients. The aim of the psychological treatment is to assist the patients to exercise their freedom and to fulfil their obligations. This primary aim is not subject to any scientific-theoretical consideration. Although Spitz and Bowlby have investigated the effects of maternal deprivation on children, these writers did not discover any new form of therapy based on a refutable theory, they simply confirmed the fact which had been known since time immemorial that babies need their mothers' love and they exposed the dire consequences which can follow from a neglect of this fundamental requirement.

D. Bardon and his associates ignored the fundamental difference between the libertarian and the deterministic principles. They treated the addition of the baby to the mother on a par with the addition of a drug. They compared their results with those of another author's, M. E. Martin, who had treated the same conditions without admitting the babies with their mothers to the hospital. The results of the comparison were equivocal and the authors concluded that further series of comparative studies are called for.

As in all statistical evaluations, the time factor is worked out. We thus learn 'the average length of stay was seven weeks [138]'.

When considering how human beings meet a challenge to their freedom, as in the case of the mothers confronted with their babies and their illness, time must be judged quite differently from the way it is judged when an illness is treated scientifically, for instance by a drug. In the latter case, one method, say treatment by drug A, may be found to be superior to treatment by drug B on account of producing quicker results. In the former case, on the other hand, the number of days or weeks is not relevant. The achievement of each person cannot be counted in measurable temporal units; in fact there are no such 'units', in subjective-historical time [139], every moment is different from every other from one person to the next, and even in the same person's life.

The difficulty lies in the interpretation of a psychological illness. From a deterministic point of view, illness, represented by the nosological diagnosis, is the result of certain deterministic factors, and treatment consists in adding another factor. The statistical evaluation of the treatment aims at eliminating the possibilities of a deception with regard to the efficacy of this factor. The underlying assumption is that in principle all cases of a certain illness can be expected to respond to the same treatment in the same manner.

From a libertarian point of view, an emotional illness is a condition of an individual self which interferes with the exercise of his or her freedom and is a failure to meet a challenge, to exercise freedom, to fulfil potentialities. Deterministic effective treatments, such as drugs, can make it easier for the patient to meet his challenge. Psychological treatments which consist in human relations are basically different from physical treatments, as the relationship between people is itself an expression of freedom, and no two people are alike, each experiences the relationship differently. Therefore it is a mistake to expect a sick self to respond to psychotherapy as the sick body does to the physical treatment of an inflamed lung or an inflamed appendix.

The illness of the self expresses itself in human relations, for instance in the way in which a woman loves or hates her baby. The relationship with the child is an expression of her freedom, it has its unique, meaningful character and therefore cannot be assessed statistically, as the items of a statistical assessment have no individuality.

The illness of the mind, understood in deterministic language, affects the illness of the self, understood in libertarian language, for the freedom of the self is limited by the way in which the mind is sick in a neurotic or psychotic manner. Hysterical, obsessional and schizophrenic people are disturbed in their selfhood by the illnesses of hysteria, obsessional neurosis and schizophrenia, all of which interfere with the way in which a man can meet the challenges of his life and can relate to other people.

The argument for the libertarian case is further complicated by the assumption of a biological-instinctual interpretation of maternity. Apart from the pathological-psychiatric determinism, the question of a biological-psychiatric determinism must be considered. Animals care for their young in an automatic, i.e. deterministic manner. But there is a difference. Women do not go through automatic, instinctual movements, they *act* when *they* care for their babies. In the human being there is human love which entails the exercise of freedom, the deliberate making of a relationship.

The human relationship of the emotionally sick person, who is treated with psychotherapy, is with the therapist. This relationship has also been considered deterministically. Like the two groups of mentally ill mothers, so two groups of mentally ill people suffering from neurosis, have been compared: one having no psychotherapy, the others receiving such treatment. A deterministic, statistical evaluation has shown that it makes no difference whether a therapist relates himself to the patient or not. In either case, seventy per cent of neurotic people improve within five years [140].

The authors of the five-year follow-up study made the same kind of mistake which Bardon and his co-workers made. Although there was no difference in the signs and symptoms of neurotic illness in the two groups, there was a difference in the experience of the people who comprised these groups. A psychotherapist can enable people to face their challenge in a way which lay people cannot do. (If the therapist follows the wrong principle and conveys to the patient a view which is based on a faulty deterministic foundation, he is likely to hinder the patient in his struggle for freedom.)

CONCLUSION

The neglect of the libertarian principle leads to faulty conclusions in Behavioural Psychiatry, in Social Psychiatry and in Individual Psychiatry. The wrong methodology leads to a denigration of human personalities, of patients and staff. Theoretical mistakes have thus grave practical consequences.

The faulty conception of the human person which has originated in the special realm of science has spread to the general realm of humanity. As the principle of freedom is the moral principle, its usurpation by determinism amounts to a demoralization of human beings.

The implications of a medically-orientated libertarianism will be evaluated in the next chapter. The freedom of the self will be related to its determinism and the subjective, experiential element to the objective, ethical principle. The aim will be to formulate a non-deterministic framework which can guide the therapist.

Before we leave the realm of epistemology, we have to investigate the problem of a common denominator for all scientific knowledge. In this enquiry too, we shall be guided by the Kantian Theory of Knowledge.

NOTES

[1] *General Psychopathology*, Engl. transl. Manchester University Press, 1962, p. 574.
[2] Anhang, second edition, 1922, Springer, Berlin.
[3] Engl. transl. by N. Kemp Smith, Macmillan & Co., London, 1929.
[4] See p. 46.
[5] *General Psychopathology*, p. 473.
[6] *Kant's Critique of Pure Reason*, Engl. transl. by N. Kemp Smith, Macmillan & Co., 1929, London, p. 551.
[7] ibid.

[8]   *Kant's Critique of Pure Reason*, p. 557.
[9]   ibid.
[10] ibid, p. 558.
[11] K. Jaspers, op. cit., p. 474.
[12] See p. 48.
[13] *Amer. J. of Psychiatry*, Oct. 1965, vol. 122, no. 4.
[14] ibid, p. 373.
[15] ibid, p. 372.
[16] ibid, p. 375.
[17] ibid, p. 374.
[18] ibid, p. 373.
[19] ibid.
[20] ibid, p. 374.
[21] *Critique of Pure Reason*, transl. by N. Kemp Smith, Macmillan & Co., 1929, London, p. 551.
[22] 'Functional Psychoses and Social Status', *Brit. J. Psychiat.* (1968), 114, pp. 733-7.
[23] 'Social Psychiatry of a Mobile Suburb', *Int. Journ. of Soc. Psych.*, Summer 1960, vol. 6, nos. 1 & 2.
[24] 'Hypochondriasis in Oriental Jewish Immigrants', *Int. J. of Soc. Psych.*, Summer 1958, vol. 4, no. 1, pp. 18-23.
[25] *The Structure of Science*, 1961, London, Routledge & Kegan Paul, Harcourt, Brace & World, U.S.A., p. 462.
[26] Leff, Julian, 1978, 'Social Psychiatry' *Brit. J. Psychiat.*, 132, p. 517.
[27] *The Structure of Science*, 1961, London, Routledge & Kegan Paul, Harcourt, Brace & World, U.S.A., pp. 468, 469.
[28] 'The Problem of Ego Identity', *J. of Americ. Psychoanalyt. Ass.*, vol. 4, 1956, p. 57.
[29] *Between Man and Man*, 1947, Kegan Paul, London, p. 203.
[30] 1967, paperback edition, Methuen & Co.
[31] ibid, p. 228.
[32] *On Agression*, Konrad Lorenz, 1967, paperback edition, Methuen & Co., p. 202.
[33] *Review of Evolutionary Ethics*, by Julian S. Huxley, Oxford University Press, published in *Mind*, vol. 53, 1944, p. 366.
[34] W. W. Norton & Co. Inc., 1953, New York.
[35] ibid, p. 5.
[36] *The Interpersonal Theory of Psychiatry*, Harry Stack Sullivan, 1953, W. W. Norton & Co. Inc., New York, p. 133.
[37] *The Structure of Science*, Routledge & Kegan Paul, 1961, p. 532.
[38] Charles C. Thomas, Springfield, Illinois, U.S.A., 1958.
[39] ibid, p. 55.
[40] ibid.

[41] ibid, p. 52.

[42] ibid, p. 69.

[43] ibid, pp. 44, 45.

[44] Jones, Maxwell, 1968, *Social Psychiatry in Practice*, The Idea of the Therapeutic Community, Harmondsworth, Penguin, pp. 30, 101.

[45] *Inmanuel Kant's Critique of Pure Reason*, transl. by Norman Kemp Smith , 1929, London, Macmillan & Co., p. 551.

[46] ibid, p. 614.

[47] *Gesammelte Schriften*, V. Band, Teubner, Leipzig, Berlin, 1924.

[48] ibid, p. 318; translation by H. A. Hodges, *Wilhelm Dilthey*, London, 1944, Kegan Paul, Trench, Trubner & Co., p. 126.

[49] Appendix in Ernest Jones, *Sigmund Freud, Life and Work*, 1955, London, The Hogarth Press, vol. 2, p. 488.

[50] *An Essay on Man*, 1944, New Haven, Yale University Press, p. 21.

[51] ibid, p. 35.

[52] *General Psychopathology*, transl. from German, 7th edition, 1963, Manchester University Press, p. 331.

[53] See for instance O. Fenichel, *The Psychoanalytic Theory of Neurosis*, Kegan Paul, Trench, Trubner & Co., London and W. W. Norton & Co., New York, 1945, pp. 4,5: 'Freud investigated the mental world in the same scientific spirit as his teachers had investigated the physical world. . . . The general laws that are valid for life phenomena are also valid for mental phenomena; special laws that are valid only for the level of mental phenomena must be added'.

[54] S. Freud, *Civilization and its Discontents*, Hogarth Press, 3rd edition, 1946, p. 102.

[55] London, 1940, Kegan Paul, Trench, Trubner & Co.

[56] ibid, p. 123.

[57] ibid, p. 124.

[58] ibid.

[59] Of course, Mannheim's sociological framework is not absolute, the individual person is not completely determined by his *milieu*.

[60] H. Guntrip, *Personality Structure and Human Interaction*, 1961, London, The Hogarth Press and the Institute of Psycho-Analysis, p. 85.

[61] *Psychoanalytic Studies of the Personality*, Tavistock/Routledge, 1952, London, p. 82.

[62] ibid, pp. 250, 251.

[63] *Psychoanalytic Studies of the Personality*, p. 53.

[64] *The Psychoanalytic Theory of Neurosis*, O. Fenichel, 1945, London, Kegan Paul, Trench, Trubner & Co., and W. W. Norton & Co., New York, p. 64.

[65] ibid, p. 5.

[66] 'Freedom and Causality', 1959, *Philosophy*, vol. 34, no. 130.

[67] ibid, p. 199.

[68] 1956, New York, Basic Books.

[69] ibid, p. 92.

[70] See p. 16.

[71] A. Adler: *Social Interest: A Challenge to Mankind*, 1938, Faber & Faber, Ltd., p. 88.

[72] ibid, p. 275.

[73] ibid, p. 273.

[74] ibid, p. 274.

[75] H. L. Ansbacher and R. R. Ansbacher, *The Individual Psychology of Alfred Adler*, 1956, New York, Basic Books, p. 175.

[76] ibid, p. 195.

[77] George Allen & Unwin, 1950, London.

[78] ibid, p. 71.

[79] 'Ist Indivualpsychologie als Wissenschaft möglich?', *Zeitschrift für Individual-psychologie*, 1914, Bd. 1, Heft 1.

[80] *The Psychology of C. G. Jung*, Engl. transl. London, 1946, Kegan Paul, Trench, Trubner & Co., p. 61.

[81] C. G. Jung, *Memories, Dreams, Reflections*, recorded and edited by Aniele Jaffe, Engl. transl. Collins, Routledge and Kegan Paul, London, 1963, p. 309.

[82] C. G. Jung, *Memories, Dreams, Reflections*, paperback, Collins, The Fontana Library. 1961, p. 160.

[83] 'Biological Theory and The Concept of Archetypes', reprinted in *New Developments in Analytical Psychology*, Routledge & Kegan Paul, London, 1957.

[84] ibid, p. 1.

[85] ibid, p. 11.

[86] ibid.

[87] ibid, p. 18.

[88] Michael Fordham, 'Reflections on Image and Symbol', reprinted in *New Developments in Analytical Psychology*, Routledge & Kegan Paul, London, 1957, p. 52.

[89] ibid.

[90] ibid, p. 60.

[91] Jolande Jacobi, *The Psychology of C. G. Jung*, London, 1946, 4th edition, Kegan Paul, Trench, Trubner & Co., p. 92.

[92] Michael Fordham, 'Reflections on Image and Symbol', p. 55.

[93] Gerhard Adler, *Studies in Analytical Psychology*, Routledge & Kegan Paul, London, 1948, p. 49.

[94] 'Reflections on the Archetypes and Synchronicity', reprinted in *New Developments in Analytical Psychology*, Routledge and Kegan Paul, London, 1957, p. 44.

[95] Michael Fordham, *The Origins of the Ego in Childhood*, ibid, p. 112.

[96] Gerhard Adler, *Studies in Analytical Psychology*, Routledge & Kegan Paul, London, 1948, p. 146.

[97] Jolande Jacobi, *The Psychology of C. G. Jung*, London, 4th edition, 1946, Kegan Paul, Trench, Trubner & Co., p. 129.

[98] 'Jung's "Archetypes" and Psychiatry', *Journ. of Mental Science* (1960), vol. 106, no. 445, p. 1518.

[99] ibid, p. 1522.

[100] C. G. Jung, *Instinct and the Unconscious, Contributions to Analytical Psychology*, Kegan Paul, Trench, Trubner & Co., 1928, p. 276.

[101] Karl Jaspers, *General Psychopathology*, transl. from the German 7th edition, 1962, Manchester University Press, p. 333.

[102] ibid.

[103] ibid.

[104] Michael Fordham, 'Biological Theory and the Concept of Archetypes', reprinted in *New Developments in Analytical Psychology*, Routledge & Kegan Paul, London, 1957, p. 9.

[105] op. cit., p. 339,

[106] In *Contributions to Analytical Psychology*, Kegan Paul, London, 1928, p. 61.

[107] 'Biological Theory and the Concept of Archetypes', op. cit., p. 17.

[108] There are innumerable ways of speculating about the psyche. Such systems of thought may well be consistent within themselves and therefore satisfactory from the logical and analytical points of view, but they cannot be put to a test which would satisfy the standards of science. Their application to emotional problems reveals their arbitrariness.

[109] 'The Chemical Theory of Temperament Applied to Introversion and Extraversion', *J. abn. soc. Psychol.*, 1929, 24, pp. 293-309.

[110] Frieda Fordham, *An Introduction to Jung's Psychology*, A Pelican Book, 1953, Penguin Books Ltd., pp. 29, 30.

[111] (1960a) *Arch. general Psychiatry*, 2, 263; and (1962) *Am. N.Y. Acad. Sc.*, 96, 438.

[112] *Brit. J. Psychiat.* (1963), 109, 231-4.

[113] *The Integration of the Personality* (1940), London, Kegan Paul, Trench, Trubner & Co., p. 25.

[114] O. Fenichel, *The Psychoanalytic Theory of Neurosis*, 1945, W. W. Norton & Co., New York, and London, Kegan Paul, Trench, Trubner & Co., p. 417.

[115] *General Psychopathology*, transl. from the German 7th edition, Manchester University Press, 1962, p. 428.

[116] *The Explanation of Behaviour*, 1964, London, Routledge & Kegan Paul; New York: The Humanities Press, p. 55.

[117] ibid.

[118] ibid.

[119] ibid, p. 56.

[120] ibid, p. 32,

[121] ibid, p. 56.

[122] Second edition, edited by E. P. Hollander and R. G. Hunt, New York Oxford University Press, London, Toronto, 1967.

[123] *Traditional Personality Theory in the Light of Recent Evidence*, ibid, pp. 136, 137.

[124] *The Explanation of Behaviour*, 1964, Routledge & Kegan Paul, New York: The Humanities Press, pp. 11, 12, 17.

[125] J. McVicker Hunt, *Traditional Personality Theory in the Light of Recent Evidence*, op. cit., p. 137.

[126] *Current Perspectives in Social Psychology*, 2nd edition, pp. 53-60.

[127] ibid, p. 54.

[128] ibid, p. 5.

[129] ibid, pp. 56, 57.

[130] ibid, p. 57.

[131] ibid, p. 56.

[132] ibid, p. 55.

[133] ibid, p. 56.

[134] Attempts directed at establishing a form of determinism which is based on the functioning of the mind without reference to the investigator's mind have led to a theory of 'functional determinism'. These attempts have failed, as the 'functional' theory presupposes a persistence of the 'social' mind which cannot be proved to exist or of a mind which is considered simply as a system of variables like a physical system which is a purely formal speculation. For the critique of functionalism see for instance E. Nagel, *The Structure of Science*, 1961, London, Routledge & Kegan Paul, pp. 520-35.

[135] 'Mother and Baby Unit: Psychiatric Survey of 115 Cases', *Brit. Med. J.*, 1968, vol. 2, pp. 775-8.

[136] ibid, p. 756.

[137] ibid.

[138] ibid, p. 758.

[139] See previous discussion on p. 82.

[140] R. Giel, R. S. Knox, C. M. Carstairs, 'A Five-year Follow-up of 100 Neurotic Out-patients', *Brit. Med. J.*, vol. 2, 1964, pp. 160-3.

PART III

Kantian Epistemology and the Unification of Scientific Thought

Man always searches for *one* principle to guide him, a universal which can explain all particulars. While his gaze is directed towards the world around him, towards the multiplicity of its contents, he postulates a metaphysical entity as their unifying basis; as a scientist, engaged in the particular study of physics, biology, psychology or any other discipline, he is tempted to claim that the concepts and principles of his particular science can serve as this unifying basis for all scientific phenomena. (As the next step he tries to annex also the domain of ethics, but the critique of this attempt will be reserved for the following chapter.) This tendency leads him from physics to physicalism, from biology to biologism and from psychology to psychologism.

Physicalism is another term for materialism, a metaphysical doctrine. Bertrand Russell, exemplifying the physicalist outlook, maintains that 'the progress of biology, physiology and psychology has made it more probable than it ever was before that all natural phenomena are governed by the laws of physics [1]'. We can agree that living bodies are made of a substance which can be subjected to physical investigations and that mental processes can be influenced by physical agents such as drugs. Bertrand Russell does not, however, mean this. He maintains that the laws of physics will probably be found sufficient to account for all phenomena, including those dealt with by biology and psychology. This attempt of physics to usurp the territory of the other sciences has led to a prejudice: the progress of science lies in physics alone.

J. H. Woodger has drawn attention to the confusion between 'applicability' of physics (and chemistry) to biology (and psychology) and 'reducibility' of one science to another [2]. The *method* of physics (and chemistry) can be used to investigate and influence biological and psychological phenomena, 'but people are not content to remain within the safe confines of methodology. Most people are natural meta-physicians, and it is an easy passage for them from the unassailable, methodological doctrine, that physics and chemistry are applicable to biological objects, to the metaphysical doctrine that living organisms are nothing but physical systems [3]'. Woodger deplores this confusion, as it 'engenders a feeling of inferiority in biologists' and 'thus retards the search for explanatory hypotheses on the biological level [4]'. Speaking as a biologist he justly protests against this form of metaphysics, which has already been discussed in the first chapter. The modern scientist and scientifically minded layman may be inclined to brush aside the notion put forward in this book and especially in the present chapter that biological and psychological phenomena are not reducible to physical phenomena, and may think that a conception of life and mind as distinct from inert matter is a retrograde step, hindering the progress of science, or a mystical belief; but the opposite is in fact the case. Science cannot develop without such insight. The recent attempts directed at creating life out of inanimate matter which have already been mentioned (Note [33], p. 61) do not affect the division of physics and biology as two distinct sciences. True, it is possible that physical processes give rise to biological phenomena, but the characteristics of these phenomena would still have to be understood as being fundamentally different from the elements from which they have arisen.

Another attempt at unification of scientific thought is *biologism*. This doctrine maintains that biology is primary and that all scientific phenomena can be deduced from it. The German biologist Adolf Meyer was of this opinion and maintained that 'physical reality is no more than a simpler model of the organic reality [5]'. In fact, he held, that 'it is the ultimate task of theoretical biology to formulate biological axioms, principles and laws, so that it would be possible to deduce from them physical laws, etc. by simplifying deduction [6]'.

Biologism not only tries to annex physics, it also claims psychology as its victim. We met such an attempt in behaviourism. Biologism is open to the same objections as physicalism.

We now come to the position taken up by those psychologists who, from their limited field, invade the rest of science and of ethics. As they operate with biological and psychological concepts, their 'ism' is mixed; it can be called *biolo-psychologism*.

Freud is an example. He started as a neurologist and never fully overcame his neurological-biological bias. He conceived mental life as analogous to physical phenomena, picturing the mind, as we saw, as an apparatus discharging libidinal energy. E. Jones, Freud's great admirer and biographer, agrees that Freud's model was constructed on physiological lines [7]. Guntrip, a neo-Freudian, refers to 'Freud's tremendous emotional struggle to transcend the categories of neurophysiology in his psychological investigations [8]'. The same author points out that 'the pleasure principle is, strictly speaking, a physiological, not a psychological, concept [9]'.

Guntrip has introduced non-biological concepts into the theory of psycho-analysis, but has not confined himself to the mental sphere; he has in fact added the psychological 'ism' to the biological doctrine. A new dynamis is envisaged: one of object exciting or rejecting. From this basis an attack is launched on the territory of sociology. The political, economic and cultural situation is seen in terms of personal relations, as an extension of the original libidinal relationship between the baby and the mother's breast. Thus, it is claimed, 'the instincts are the prime movers of all human activity [10]', a view held originally by McDougall and in line with biolo-psychologism. Instinct is, however, a biological concept and cannot explain those aspects of social life in which economic, cultural and historical factors play a fundamental part. Relationships between people cannot be reduced to an instinctual level (this usurpation concerns ethics and will be discussed further in the next chapter). Biologo-psychologism, like the other 'isms' falls into error and confusion. Scientific knowledge cannot be unified by one particular scientific system which in its confines cannot absorb the whole field of knowledge, incorporating ethics as well.

A different attempt at the unification of scientific knowledge, not based on one particular discipline, is made by the philosophy of nominalism. All sciences deal with the general as distinct from the particular, i.e. with 'universals'. They are the names of objects and their properties, the symbols, the purely formal aspect.

The nominalist is concerned solely with the meanings of words, with semantics, with the terms which are employed in science and with the role of scientific abstraction. Crookshank has applied this principle to medicine and has pointed out that the term 'disease' is a universal which must not be hypostatized, i.e. made into an entity [11]. The purely nominalistic approach is, however, insufficient in the end; for it misses out the substance to which the term refers.

As an illustration, take the term 'pleurisy'. It refers to certain changes in the organ called the pleura, but the use of the term also implies the acceptance of the notion that there is a body which can be divided into parts and of the theory that changes of a particular kind are explained as being due to the invasion of micro-organisms. 'Pleurisy' is thus a universal, but it can be understood only with reference to the reality of the concrete body (which, however, cannot be known as such) and a particular abstract medical theory of bodily illness. The same considerations which hold good for pleurisy apply to other diseases.

The nominalistic approach has been developed in biology by J. H. Woodger. He distinguishes two attitudes towards scientific knowledge: one which understands science 'as a system of rules for manipulating the things we find in the world' and another which 'understands it as a metaphysical doctrine about a world behind the scenes of ordinary life [12]'. We need not quarrel over the rejection of the second alternative, as the world as such in unknowable: we have to find out what is involved in the first interpretation and whether no third possibility exists.

Woodger calls himself a nominalist, i.e. he is concerned with language, in science with records. He starts with observation records and stresses the fact that these can be generalized. He mentions the example of William Harvey's theory of the circulation of the blood and, in particular, his observation that the contraction of the heart is followed by a dilation of the arteries. The subsequent universal statement is quoted by Woodger as follows: 'Whenever the heart is in systole the arteries are in diastole [13]'. These observation records are called also 'zero-level hypotheses'. Then a new unifying idea is introduced through the 'explanatory hypotheses' which shows a much wider spread of consequences than the generalization or zero-level hypotheses which it was introduced to cover [14]'. The latter have certain consequences. All these should remain within one particular science and not enter the field of another. This is violated in the case of a mixed neurological and psychological language.

Woodger maintains that he can derive consequences from the scientist's statements without reference to their meaning by using 'formative' signs, a term introduced by K. R. Popper in a paper entitled 'Logic without Assumptions [15]'. He uses a mathematical procedure which was introduced during the last century by two mathematicians, Boole and Frege. Herein lies the nominalistic aspect of his method [16].

The method has not been generally accepted by biologists and experts have criticized this application of the mathematical theory. This issue must be judged by those who have the necessary knowledge. We are not concerned with this question, but with the role of nominalism in science. Woodger leaves his reader in no doubt that 'the procedure of natural science begins and ends with observations [17]'. He stresses the need for the 'bright idea' which inspires the scientist who then has to check his new theory by observations. This flight of the imagination is not formal-nominalistic.

According to Woodger theoretical thought can proceed without reference to the nature of the phenomena concerned on a purely formal basis. This is the case in physics where the theory is formulated in mathematical symbols; in chemistry a formal approach has been able to determine the characteristics of certain elements through the framework of the periodic system before they had been discovered. In medicine, such procedure is available only in exceptional cases. It is possible to calculate the chances of an inherited characteristic appearing amongst a number of children if its general genetic pattern is known. There is no need here to refer to the nature of the particular phenomenon. Even in these cases, the phenomena are, however, not named arbitrarily and the theories dealing with them are not divorced from their material.

Generally speaking, theories can be developed in medicine only in close touch with experiment and observation, and not on formal lines. The designations of diseases are not arbitrary and medical science is not suspended in a void. The terminology of medicine is not a matter of agreeing on a definition without reference to the material with which doctors are dealing, namely sick people. The names of diseases could not be changed like the names of chessmen where such a change would not destroy the game. Therefore nominalism cannot be the unifying principle in medicine.

In order to attain a point of view which unifies scientific thought, the scientist must learn to turn his glance away from the objects of nature, from what is usually called 'reality', which is unknowable. While he naively believes that he can obtain knowledge by simply observing objects which he perceives with his senses or while he hypostatizes concepts (i.e. makes them into objects), any valid unification is impossible. The scientist has to learn to look at the source of scientific knowledge, which is the *mind*. He must fully realize that science is abstract, built up of abstract concepts which form theories. He must understand the tools which his mind uses in the creation of science.

The man who undertakes research in the field of science must examine his equipment even more carefully than the man who builds a house because the scientist's tools are more important for his work than the builder's for his job. Even if the hammer and the chisel are of poor quality, the bricks and mortar, the material structure of the house, do not suffer. The tools of the scientist, unlike those of the builder, form part of the structure of the building itself. The tools are the concept with which the mind builds up the particular science. If the wrong (metaphysical) concepts are used, or if one science forces its concepts on another for which they are unsuitable, the whole building becomes unsound.

Physics and chemistry enter into medicine in so far as the body can be analysed into elements which obey the laws of these sciences. The analytical approach follows the principle of mechanistic materialism. Biology is, however, the science of the living organism; it also makes use of the analytical mechanistic-materialistic method, but can deal with the teleological (holistic) feature of life only by comparing it with human motivation, which means that life is inscrutable. Psychology cannot be formulated as a science of the whole psyche, there are only detailed psychological assessments of certain psychic phenomena.

The scientist who has gone through the 'Copernican Revolution' avoids the mistakes to which the naive realist is prone. He recognizes the situation in each science and respects its individuality. He will also respect ethics and not try to submerge it in the realm of deterministic science. He has found the true common denominator which unites scientific knowledge.

NOTES

[1] *The Scientific Outlook,* Allen & Unwin, 1931, p. 125.
[2] *Biology and Language,* Cambridge University Press, 1952, p. 338.
[3] ibid, p. 336.
[4] ibid.
[5] *Ideen und Ideale biologischer Erkenntnis,* Joh. Ambrosius Barth, Leipzig, 1934, p. 37.
[6] ibid, p. 49.
[7] See H. Guntrip, *Personality Structure and Human Interaction,* The Hogarth Press and the Institute of Psychoanalysis, 1961, p. 120.
[8] ibid, p. 122.
[9] ibid, p. 126.
[10] ibid, p. 260.
[11] C. K. Ogden and I. A. Richards, *The Meaning of Meaning,* II. Supplement, Kegan Paul, Trench, Trubner & Co., 1936, p. 346.
[12] *Physics, Psychology and Medicine, a Methodological Essay,* Cambridge University Press, 1956, p. 12.
[13] ibid, p. 16.
[14] ibid, p. 19.
[15] *Proc. Aristotelean Soc.,* 5 May 1947, pp. 251-92.

[16] *Biology and Language,* Cambridge University Press, 1952.
[17] *Physics, Psychology and Medicine,* Cambridge University Press, 1956, p. 36.

CHAPTER III

Medicine and Ethics

Medicine and Ethics

INTRODUCTION

In the previous chapters, the patient was considered as an object of science, and although views were also expressed about the patient as a person, as a subject, no attempt was made to formulate in detail the ethical issues raised by this distinction or to describe their significance for medicine. It is to this task that we now must turn.

Man is a free being, which means that he is able to choose and to make decisions. He has, further, a conscience which makes him aware of his duties towards himself and others, of potentials which he must try to realize and obligations which he must try to fulfil. Life, for him, is experienced as a challenge and he feels guilty when he fails to meet this challenge.

The doctor's position with regard to his patient's values and moral views is frequently and unfortunately neglected in medical education. Of course, a doctor's position in relation to his patient as a moral being is different from that of a judge or priest. They pronounce on what is right or wrong, the judge in the name of the law, the priest in the name of God. A doctor, naturally, has no such authority and cannot in his medical role act as judge in regard to a patient's morals.

The patient is his own judge, however. His conscience tells him if he has adopted the wrong values and has thereby missed opportunities in his life. As a result of having failed in such ways, he is liable to feel ill, becoming anxious and depressed; he may then give up the struggle and withdraw or even attempt to take his life. In such cases, the doctor's help is needed. Thus ethics cannot be excluded from medicine.

While ethical problems inevitably confront him, however, the doctor's role remains different from that of the moral philosopher. The latter's concern is theoretical: he is interested in formulating a theory consistent in itself, in which 'good' and 'bad' figure as predicates. The doctor's concern is practical: the treatment of sickness or its prevention. For these purposes the doctor has to understand the effects which different moral views may have on a person's attitude and conduct: he has to enable his patient to recognize the significance of these views for him and he must be ready tb help the patient to alter his perspective if it is detrimental, and if the patient is prepared to adopt a better set of values. At the same time, however, the doctor must avoid imposing his own values on his patient. To aid him in this difficult, but necessary endeavour, he needs to have some awareness of the effects of unexamined presuppositions in the fields both of ethical theory and of scientific knowledge.

The type of moral philosophy which a doctor is likely to have adopted without being aware of it, is naturalistic ethics. This is an obvious consequence of the predominance of naturalistic science in his medical education. The naturalistic viewpoint holds that such moral attributes as 'good', 'right' and 'wrong' can be completely analysed in terms of non-moral predicates, e.g. libidinal satisfaction and dissatisfaction.

MEDICINE AND NATURALISTIC ETHICS – THE PATIENT AS OBJECT

Some of the moral implications of the naturalistic viewpoint were mentioned at the end of the last chapter. We must now consider the consequences for the patient of the infringement of science on the moral sphere, a phenomenon which can be termed 'scientism'. We consider first the effects of scientific treatment on the patient who is considered to be merely an object of science.

As we have seen, mechanistic materialism is the hallmark of science. This means that phenomena are regarded as devoid of individuality and that the whole is conceived as consisting of isolated units, their common ground being the self-identical substrate. Patients, treated as 'material' for scientific purposes (such as research) on mechanistic-materialistic lines, lose their individuality in the doctor's eyes: they become bearers of a disease. In the statistical evaluation the individual with his uniqueness gets lost.

There has been much complaint recently about the effects of such treatment and medical authorities have gradually become aware of this incursion of science into ethics. One of them, N. Morris, has written of the effect of this 'scientific' attitude upon women in labour [1]. Morris has described how the woman is made into the material which the hospital staff expect. He states that 'many of our present procedures, which involve dragooning and regimentation, must be revised [2]'. He disapproves of a form of classifying patients which is not dictated by the requirements of scientific systematization but by the need to produce willing clinical material. 'We must get rid of that awful method of dividing patients into "co-operative" or "unco-operative", into "easy" or "difficult" '. He writes: 'This classification is largely based on how much regimentation the patient will stand without complaining [3]'. It must be admitted that there are hostile, often unconscious, feelings in the minds of doctors and nurses involved, but apart from these, the indifference of the purely scientifically-minded doctor towards his patients is unethical. The patient is more than an object of science.

We saw that mechanistic materialism assumes that phenomena occur in an unbroken chain of cause and effect. In medicine, the patient is studied by different sciences, each utilizing a deterministic approach and conceiving him to be the result of the different factors: genetic, biological, biochemical, biophysical, sociological, cultural and historical. The scientific approach can reveal to what extent men are actually determined by factors beyond their control, but men are also free beings. By not respecting a patient's freedom, a doctor conveys to the patient the feeling of being fated. This leads to despondency and hopelessness in those cases where the doctor cannot remove the cause of the disease, as in neurotic illness. As a result, the patient does not make the necessary effort to help himself. In physical illness, the same attitude of resignation is responsible for lack of co-operation in the treatment and for the enormous waste of opportunities in the field of preventing illness by healthier living. Doctors have conveyed to their patients and to the population at large the idea that they, as lay people, are not responsible for their own health, that health and disease are a matter to which only scientifically-trained doctors can attend. The population swallow pills, submit to injections and to operations without having any idea what is happening to their bodies and minds under such treatment. They are the objects of deterministic science and not free people using their own intelligence.

The medical profession in Great Britain have recently become aware of the need for public health education. As the *British Medical Journal* points out, 'medical men are aware of the frustration that their therapeutic efforts are apt to meet because patients will not, or cannot, relinquish unhealthy habits. Adult men and women smoke their way into lung cancer, bronchitis, and coronary disease . . . [4]'. We learn from the same article that in 1959 the Central and Scottish Health Services Council was set up to look after health education.

Education implies appealing to the free will of the person who is to be educated, and it is therefore important that the educator give the right example by acting with the responsibility which he expects from those whom he tries to educate. This principle is not fulfilled by those doctors who kill themselves or ruin their health through smoking cigarettes [5].

The doctor can thus be defeated in his therapeutic efforts through failing to see his patient as a person, i.e. by acting only as a scientist. The faults of such a philosophy of medicine become even more serious in the practices of medical psychologists who sacrifice the idea of freedom to the deterministic approach of their particular school.

Deterministic Psychologies

Medical psychology was examined from an epistemological point of view in the last chapter. It was found that its theories necessarily differed from those of physics and biology: each school was shown to be lacking in a scientific theoretical framework and to be indulging in metaphysical statements about the nature of man. It was pointed out that, as a result of its deterministic orientation, such treatment was ethically unsound and harmful. A more detailed examination of the harmful effects of these treatments is now in order.

(a) BEHAVIOUR THERAPY

The different applications of behaviour therapy have already been described and criticized from an epistemological point of view. From an ethical point of view, it is important to realize that behaviour therapists in general tend to deny or neglect the existence of a mind from which the illness originates (this criticism does not contradict the thesis that the mind is not a scientific concept; we are dealing here with the patient's feeling of having or of not having a mind). Behaviour therapists isolate learning processes and consider them to be the responses to stimuli. In their treatment, they set new stimuli ʹ work to produce 'more appropriate' responses.

As behaviour therapists in common with other psychotherapists publish only those cases which have been successful and do not give details of the cases in which they have failed, it is necessary to illustrate the criticism by citing a 'successful' case, and suggesting that the interpretation was wrong and may have been harmful.

The case, selected from the literature of behaviour therapy, concerns a little girl who was treated because she had refused to eat. The symptom had appeared after her father's death. 'The therapist adopted the father's role in a variety of circumstances, ranging in order from play with dolls' tea-sets to the actual eating situation, and reinforced

those reactions which were considered desirable. The theoretical rationale was that the father had become a conditioned stimulus on which
eating depended [6]'. The rationale does not appear creditable to
anyone not previously committed to the schematic determinism of
behaviourist therapy. It is obvious that the father was not just 'a conditioned stimulus on which eating depended' but was a loved person
whom she was mourning. Her refusal of food was an expression of a
grief which had affected her whole soul. The favourable result was due
to the fact that a new 'father' had appeared who played with her as her
father had done. The recovery would not have been effected or would
have been followed by a relapse and even a more serious breakdown of
her personality if she had realized that the therapist had no feelings for
her, but simply went through the motions of treatment to set up new
'stimuli'.

The behaviourist is led to his denial of love by the deterministic
framework which is characteristic of scientism. The resulting confusion
is liable to cause harm to the patient's sense of values and might in
some circumstances cause further signs and symptoms of illness.

(b) FREUDIAN PSYCHOLOGY

Whereas in behaviour therapy the father is not an object of love but a
'conditioned stimulus', Freudian psychology recognizes love as a feeling
but interprets it in its own naturalistic way. Psycho-analysis was criticized in the last chapter for its dogmatic, metaphysical character, and
for its reduction of men to the biological level. As Ernest Jones wrote,
Freud 'could find no evidence of any instinct impelling man towards
higher moral, ethical or spiritual aims [7]'. The lack of such findings
results from scientism, from the instinctual theory; for 'higher moral,
ethical, or spiritual aims' are certainly not the domain of 'impelling
instincts'. Jones tells us that Freud called the idea of these aims a
'benevolent illusion [8]'. True to the viewpoint of naturalistic ethics,
psycho-analysis ignores the moral character of man and converts moral
into non-moral phenomena: Hence we have the following Freudian
statement: 'The present development of human beings requires, as it
seems to me, no different explanation from that of animals. What
appears in a minority of human individuals as an untiring impulsion
towards further perfection can easily be understood as a result of the
instinctual repression upon which is based all the most precious in
human civilization [9]'.

Freud's conception of love follows from his instinctual conception
of man: 'The nucleus of what we mean by love naturally consists (and
this is what is commonly called love, and what the poets sing of) in

sexual love with sexual union as its aim. But we do not separate from this – what in any case has a share in the name "love". – on the one hand self love, and on the other, love for parents and children, friendship and love for humanity in general and also devotion to concrete objects and to abstract ideas [10]'. Freud justifies this contention by referring to his researches. The argument is not valid, however, as it is circular: there is only instinctual libido in Freud's naturalistic system. The importance of sexual relationship is not to be denied, but what must be denied is the role which the Freudian attaches to it as a primary fundamental force. Difficulties within a marriage, for instance, may well include sexual disharmony, but the underlying trouble is frequently lack of non-sexual maturity of the people concerned, leading to lack of sympathy, of kindliness, manliness, etc. These are not primarily sexual attributes. Impotence and frigidity and other obvious sexual difficulties arise from the failure of confidence, and of communication between the partners. Sexual perversions are also not primarily libidinal disturbances but are the results of weak father figures or lack of love from a mother. Identification which Freud recognized as an important factor is not a libidinal process, but is the result of feeling admiration for the particular person. Admiration is admiration of his strength, his whole personality, his moral qualities. A patient who is given the idea that all such emotions are sexual and that his disturbance is due to a biological-instinctual disturbance is thereby misled and suffers damage to his sense of values as a result.

Freud's theory also confuses the patient in regard to other matters which are not sexual. Let us consider the view taken of a child's love for his parents. According to Freud the child in the Oedipus situation 'has found the first object for his love in one or other of his parents, and all of his sexual instincts with their demand for satisfaction have been united upon this object [11]'. The sexual instinct is then 'inhibited', but ' "sensual" tendencies remain more or less strongly preserved in the unconscious, so that in a certain sense the whole of the original current continued to exist [12]'. In an analysis, these feelings are brought into the conscious mind. The patient may be made to face the sexual element in his relations with his parents, which certainly does exist, but he will be deprived of the non-sexual feelings of unselfish love, of faith and trust in his relationship with his parents, which also exist, but for which there is no room in the biologically-orientated system of psycho-analysis. This is a serious loss to him.

Further shocks await the patient. His parent does not remain the object of an instinctual urge, but is presented to him as super-ego, as conscience. As such, the parent makes demands to check the child's instinctual desire and threatens punishment should the check fail. The child thus lives in continuous fear of being deprived of the parent's affection.

It is not denied that parents implant authoritarian conscience in their children's minds, but this 'conscience' must not be confused with conscience as such, as Freud does. For, 'the prescriptions of authoritarian conscience are not determined by one's own value judgment [as those of genuine conscience are] but exclusively by the fact that its commands and tabus are pronounced by authorities. If these norms happen to be good, conscience will guide man's action in the direction of the good ... If they are bad, they are just as much part of conscience [13]'. The patient feels that he is entirely dependent on the external or internalized authority; it has to be pleased, otherwise he feels guilty. The patient is given the idea that, with such a parent, he has no right to question or to criticize the authority which has complete superiority. The bearer of the 'moral' principle thus becomes the bearer of demoralization.

There is, in addition, an emphasis on internalized cultural conscience which is conceived as a force by the aid of which society suppresses the original and primary aggressive instinct of the individual. Freud held that the individual has to pay for this suppression by neurotic illness. Again we have to admit that such tyranny exists. 'Overt authority has been replaced by anonymous authority, overt commands by "scientifically" established formulas, "don't do this", by "you will not like to do this" [14]'. The author of these words, Erich Fromm, maintains that 'the scars left from the child's defeat in the fight against irrational authority are to be found at the bottom of every neurosis [15]'. He describes vividly how the self is weakened and substituted by a pseudo-self which becomes 'the sum total of others' expectations [16]'.

The remedy for the patient who has realized the disastrous effects of the authoritarian super-ego would seem to lie in awakening in him that conscience which is not the internalized authority of parents or society. He would then be given back his human dignity and made to experience his freedom and his responsibility to choose as his conscience requires. Unfortunately, Freudian psychology is prevented by its very conception of conscience from performing this most necessary service. This attitude towards values, which entails serious negative consequences for the patient's outlook on life, follows directly from the instinctual basis of Freudian psychology.

Man is pictured basically as striving for pleasure which is achieved when instinct is gratified. Such striving and pleasure can, of course, not be denied and many aspects of life can be explained in this way. As a general outlook, hedonism is, however, sterile, as pleasure soon grows stale and turns to displeasure. The theory did not change its hedonistic character when Freud introduced the 'reality principle', as he did not think of this as something which man had to face to prove his courage, his moral fibre, but as the principle which he had to face in order to avoid loss of pleasure, which is pain. Thus the Freudian outlook of hedonism which follows from the premises of instinctual determinism is liable to make a patient unfit for the struggle of life; for life *is* a challenge, the meeting of which requires the acceptance of primary values apart from pleasure.

(c) JUNGIAN PSYCHOLOGY

Behaviour Therapy considers man in terms of stimulus and response, Freudian psychology in terms of libidinal energy, an analogue of physical energy. Both these schools are deterministic and rationalistic. Rationalistic determinism denies human freedom and thus excludes man's moral dimension. It is now necessary to examine the influence of irrational determinism on the moral sphere, as exemplified in the psychology of C. G. Jung.

The deterministic basis of Jung's psychology lies in his interpretation of myths, fairy tales, dreams and symptoms of mental illness such as delusions. The origin of these phenomena is found in the archetype, pre-existing as a form in the unconscious. Jung denied that an archetype is determined with regard to its content. 'A primordial image is determined with regard to its content only when it has become conscious and is therefore filled out with the material of conscious experience [17]'. In spite of this denial, however, the archetypes appear in Jung's writings as forces which determine a man's fate. We found (p. 90) that he called them 'the *a priori* determining constituents of all experience . . . inherited psychic qualities [18]'. They 'come upon us fatefully [19]'. Jung gives an example of the fateful activity of one archetype, the anima: 'When a highly honoured scholar in his seventies deserts his family and marries a twenty-year-old, red-haired actress, then we know that the gods have claimed another victim. It is thus that demonic supremacy shows itself to us [20]'.

Jung has denied that he is responsible for the emergence of archetypal images in his patients [21]. Such events apparently just happened to some of Jung's patients. But, surely, his interpretation of the 'events' must have been of immense significance in their appearance. If the 'honoured scholar' of the above citation was one of Jung's patients, he would have been given to understand that his fate was inevitable, whereas if he had consulted another psychiatrist, convinced of man's essential freedom, he would have been told that he was free to choose, as the old Goethe did when he fell in love with a girl of sixteen, yet did not succumb to his infatuation. It would seem that according to Jung, man's only freedom lies in learning to accept the archetypal contents of the unconscious, to be aware of them and to integrate them into his conscious mind. 'The essential thing is to differentiate oneself from these unconscious contents by personifying them and at the same time to bring them into relationship with consciousness. That is the technique of stripping them of their power [22]'. The anima is not to be trusted, she destroys people, although she gives warnings to those who ask for it. Jung did not credit a man with a great deal of freedom in his dealings with the archetypes. Under their influence man feels 'uncomfortable', 'undignified', 'unethical [23]'. Man cannot free himself from this state, however, until the right feeling comes over him [24]. Thus Jung conceived man to be determined by fate and accepted the naturalistic viewpoint; by contrast, non-naturalistic ethics holds that man is free to meet the challenge with which life presents him.

Another aspect of the inadequacy of Jungian ethics is evident in Jung's treatment of the mandala. In genuine ethics, conflicts between right and wrong are irreconcilable, but in Jungian psychology all opposites are reconciled in the mandala and the devil is given a comfortable place as an equal to God [25].

The deterministic approach which makes the archetypes into all-powerful fateful forces causes moral damage from still another viewpoint by sabotaging Jung's ethical idea of individuation, of making oneself into a 'separate, indivisible unity or whole [26]'. How can there be uniqueness and selfhood if we are the playthings of such elemental forces! 'The course of the individual human being is here as it were raised to a mere casuistic process of realisation in which the universal principle is seen in mystical contemplation [27]'. The author of these words, H. Trüb, was one of Jung's pupils and has reported an admission of the master which caused him great disappointment; said Jung: 'The personal element is for me something so irrational and accidental that I cannot do anything with it – I cannot help it, I just remove it from my sight [28]'.

Thus the value of the individual, the great ethical principle, is lost. A further loss follows in spite of Jung's denial: the loss of human relationship. Instead of being directed towards human beings, the Jungian orientation is directed towards a psychic cosmos, the forces in the unconscious. Jung himself told Trüb, who wanted to meet the world *in concreto,* that 'the way leading to - the world should not be sought because in the concept of the self the relationship with the world is already included [29]'. Thus Jung's self as archetypal self cannot express itself in a personal encounter with another self or with the world. Such a lack is of the greatest importance for patients who need personal contact and the responsibility which goes with it. With the lack of responsibility towards the individual goes the lack of social responsibility. 'Jung's private myth stirs no social trouble. This modern form of quietism is a powerful answer to the question of how to live in the modern world. It is also an answer that denies, in principle, any significant social responsibility [30]'.

Jung's elucidation of the irrational and creative aspects of the psyche and of the conflicts within its sphere remain important contributions to medical psychology which must, however, be incorporated within a different framework. Contrary to their treatment by Jung, the patient's values must not be conceived as subject to deterministic forces and powers in any total fashion.

MEDICINE AND EXISTENTIAL ETHICS – THE PATIENT AS SUBJECT

In contrast to naturalistic-deterministic ethics which ignore the patient's subjectivity and freedom, the form of ethics which doctors can accept as a guide for their practice is existential; it meets the following requirements:

(1) It is based on the affirmation of freedom and the absoluteness of conscience: moral predicates are considered to be autonomous and not to be derivable from non-moral predicates.

(2) It makes allowance for the diminution of freedom through various influences which affect the personality, especially those concerning the health of the body and the mind.

(3) It is, moreover, not a schematic moral philosophy which doctors might be tempted to impose on their patients.

In order to develop a medical approach which is existential in its ethical content, it is necessary to give up the objective standpoint of scientism and to re-discover man's subjective world. This task can be completed by utilizing the phenomenological method of Edmund Husserl; for Husserlian phenomenology brought about a revolution of thought by taking as its point of departure the data of consciousness, the subjective experiential elements of man's inner world. Husserl did not deny that an objective world or objective values existed, he 'put them into brackets', i.e. disregarded their presumed presence [31]. Husserl described his standpoint by saying: 'We fix our eyes steadily upon the sphere of consciousness and study what it is that we find immanent in *it* [32]'.

The introduction of the ethical principle into the subjective, phenomenological approach follows from the fact that man is aware of his duties towards himself and towards others, that he himself acknowledges — in principle — absolute conscience and freedom.

Existentialism which includes the phenomenological viewpoint understands human existence as grounded in freedom: to exist is 'to take leave of what one is (*ex*) in order to establish oneself (*sistere*) on the level of that which was formerly only possible [33]'. The existential philosophers are in essential agreement about the fundamental role of freedom but differ in their attitude toward the existence of a standard which can provide the criteria for choice, for the acceptance of one value in preference to another. Indeed this is but a symptom of the modern dilemma which is of such concern to existential philosophers and which is expressed as the 'death' of God.

Lacking a divinely sanctioned moral foundation, man is liable to fall prey to a feeling of despair and hopelessness, leading to the syndrome of what V. E. Frankl calls 'noogenic' neurosis. This danger is naturally of concern to the psychiatrist. It does not arise from a particular illness such as an abnormality in the patient's metabolism or from a fault in his upbringing. It is rather *'la maladie du siècle'*.

The existential psychiatrist [34] can find much elucidation of his patients' fundamental problems in the writings of the existential philosophers. He must, however, differ basically from all those writers who have claimed to know the elements of human existence as such, man's true nature. The existential psychiatrist cannot accept such claims, for to accept them and thus join the cult of a particular philosopher, would be incompatible with his scientific outlook which demands a critical mind and an attitude which is non-sectarian and which has as its only consideration the welfare of patients [35].

Apart from restricting the doctor's freedom, the acceptance of a claim that one particular philosophy represents *the* true interpretation of human existence would lead to a denial of the patient's freedom and would destroy the basis of existential psychotherapy: the ability to step out of one existence in order to establish oneself in another.

The claim of having obtained knowledge of existence conflicts not only with the ethical principle as presented in this book, but also with the epistemological principle which was laid down in the last chapter. Such knowledge would presume to be knowledge of something infinite and absolute; it would be irrefutable. Existence, i.e. Being of man as such, is unknowable: it is a metaphysical and not a scientific concept.

To deny that existential ontologies are true accounts of Being, however, does not mean that they have no truth for the person who experiences their significance in his own world. The psychiatrist can learn from the study of the different existential philosophies in what sort of worlds his patients live and can bring such understanding to bear on the therapeutic situation. 'Existential therapy attempts to bring an awareness of the manner in which the person grasps and shapes his world, and this should lead to the awareness of the availability and necessity of the ultimate existential focus, [defined as] the meaning and motivating force of a person's existence [36]'.

The Integration of the Existential and Phenomenological Principles within a Medical Framework

In order to proceed further, it is necessary to integrate the existential and phenomenological principles within a medical framework. *Phenomenology* in Husserl's sense is a description of the data of consciousness. The data compose a person's world of experience.

The existential-ethical principle is embodied in the self, the agent who is according to its own judgement responsible for behaviour, for facing life, for taking on responsibilities and for making decisions for which the person is accountable. The crucial ethical decision for the self is the choice of values which act as a guide to conduct, which is judged by the self to be right or wrong. The self therefore judges itself as if it were somebody else. This objective relation of a self to itself makes it permissible to use the term 'authentic' in describing a self, meaning thereby, an ethical person or a self which is true to itself, is genuine and thus, as far as possible is coping with the tasks of life. The self as an actual self judges itself from an ethical point of view applying to its actions and intentions the standard of an ideal self, a self towards which it strives and which it tries to establish for itself. 'A real (ideal) authentic self is something to be discovered and created, not a given, but a lifelong endeavour [37]'.

A person is conscious of his acts and intentions as moral or immoral and judges them as such. In this way the *ethical* can be seen to be clearly *related* to the *phenomenological*, conscience to consciousness.

The world in which a person lives is also judged by him from a moral point of view, and this 'world' is indeed shaped by his vision. A hedonistic ethical view for instance leads the person into a world in which considerations for pleasure play the prominent part. A puritan self, on the other hand, becomes the author of a world controlled by ideas of duty which are projected on all experience. Thus the ethical dominates the phenomenological: the world of experience is in essence (though not in fact) a reflection of the self and its moral standards.

The ethical is thus seen to be an objective, the phenomenological a subjective element in the present framework and the *medical* must now be introduced as another objective element. Medical principles provide an objective basis for judging both the world of the patient and his self, as a bearer of conscience, to be either healthy or ill. This entails recognition of the diminution of the patient's freedom in illness, which is in accord with the second requirement of an existential medical ethics [38].

Therefore what the patient experiences as his conscience, his duties and his guilt, may appear to the psychiatrist (quā doctor) to be manifestations of an illness which has caused illusions in the patient's mind and is therefore judged *medically* entirely differently from the way the patient judges himself. On the other hand, in contrast to traditional medical psychologies, the psychiatrist who accepts the existential point of view does not deny that a person can be guilty or that he has a conscience (i.e. a healthy conscience), which has not been affected by the processes of illness. The existential approach manifests itself only in its affirmation of conscience as the arbiter of right and wrong, but also in the respect which the doctor shows to the patient's world of experience, to its particular individual structure. This respect is experienced by the patient himself, thus making it possible for doctor and patient to enter into a personal relationship which is quite different from the relationship between the scientifically-minded physician and the patient who is his object of study and treatment.

Medical judgement must be used in deciding whether to employ the existential approach therapeutically, that is whether to attempt to make the patient aware of his ethical situation, his responsibilities towards himself and towards others. Even if the psychiatrist is convinced that his patient is in the throes of a moral conflict, that his symptoms stem from an existential conflict, it still does not follow that the patient should be expected under any circumstances to face this conflict: for he may be judged from the medical point of view not to possess the strength required to cope with the situation. In that case, the attempt to answer his existential challenge would only lead to a deterioration of his health and to further symptoms of a nervous breakdown. Instead, in such a case, other psychological measures must be employed which give encouragement and comfort to the patient. In addition, drugs may have to be used in order to pacify the mind, reduce tension and combat depression. Such pharmacological treatment need not be just aimed at symptoms but can be used within the fundamental existential approach, enabling the patient to cope with an otherwise overwhelming existential situation. Another measure which may be necessary either merely to reduce suffering or to enable a patient to use his freedom, is the effort to change his environment, especially the attitude of people who have dominated his self and against whom he has felt powerless. Whether the existential therapist decides to use the existential approach or not, he respects the patient in any case as an ethical person. Although he may judge him medically to be too weak to respond to the appeal to his freedom – the patient's status as a person is for him, never in question.

The introduction of non-existential therapies into the discussion raises the question of the significance of the causal principle in the deterministic and the libertarian approaches respectively.

Physical treatments, such as applications of drugs, cause an improvement in the patient's mental illness by altering his cerebral condition, whereas social treatment consisting of an alteration of the communal environment, causes relief by abolishing friction between the patient and his fellow human beings. Both therapies assume that the person has been made ill by forces which are beyond his control.

An existential personal treatment does not aim at removing any causes of illness, but expects the patient to exercise his freedom so that he himself can cause his improvement. While he must adopt a different attitude in meeting his personal challenges, existential psychotherapy is not confined to the subjective level, but accepts also the need for objectivity.

Doctor and patient both think in terms of illness as an objective event which occurs at a certain time and which represents an entity. This conception applies to mental illness such as schizophrenia or hysteria and to physical illness such as measles or rheumatoid arthritis. Such entities do not, however, fit into the phenomenological approach. Life experience is continuous, although it has its ups and downs. The 'downs', called 'illnesses', occupy certain portions of a person's life, but the character of the mental disease is often also found in the 'ups', though in a milder form. People have a general tendency to be anxious, depressed, obsessional, etc. By contrast, in the physical realm, there is a definable difference between health and disease.

The fact that emotional life is a 'flow' makes it difficult to define what constitutes a 'cure' of emotional illness. The patient may be feeling better, i.e. he may be experiencing life as less painful. He may also be able to cope better with his tasks and therefore may be improved from the phenomenological and from the existential points of view. It would, however, be wrong to say that the doctor has 'caused' the change for the better, through existential therapy, as this would imply that the patient was just an object for the doctor's treatment. It would be more correct to say that there has been some interaction between the personalities of doctor and patient, and that as the result of this communion, the improvements have come about. The doctor's part in the treatment cannot be isolated: he does not treat an illness; for 'illness' is a concept which abstracts from the experience of life. On the other hand, as a branch of psychiatric medicine, existential psychiatry must formulate a diagnostic concept of the healthy and the sick *self*.

The morally *healthy self* which is also free from symptoms of mental breakdown is the true self, the self of the authentic person; he can meet the challenges which arise in his life and can cope with his responsibilities towards himself and others. In spite of all difficulties which he may encounter he feels real, alive and whole, he experiences life as meaningful and the world as a continuum. A self owes its health to a strong constitution and to favourable conditions, especially during childhood and adolescence when it develops and matures. A secure home in which parents and children live in harmony is obviously the best environment for the development of a healthy self. Political and economic circumstances which promote the feeling of security are also important as is a general cultural climate characterized by faith in values and in their substantial truth.

By contrast, the morally *sick self* is liable to experience the symptoms of a nervous breakdown; it is the self of an inauthentic person, who cannot cope with the responsibilities of a life, such a person feels dead, unreal, and finds himself in a 'dead' and 'unreal' world which is lacking in continuity. The general symptoms which he experiences are severe anxiety and depression; these induce him to consult a psychiatrist. In them the existential psychiatrist recognizes demoralization and aims to bring about a conscious awareness in the patient of his situation and to help him to establish a healthier self.

The psychiatrist must be acquainted with the phenomenology of the demoralized self. R. D. Laing has provided an important basis for gaining the necessary insight into the phenomenology of this demoralization in his study of *The Divided Self* [39]. In this book Laing uses as a criterion for his clinical inquiry the security or insecurity of his patient's existence, for which he has chosen the adjective 'ontological' employed in an empirical sense. The above descriptions of the healthy and sick self correspond roughly to Laing's account of 'ontologically' secure and insecure people [40].

Laing describes three forms of anxiety of the 'ontologically' insecure person. They are of interest to the existential psychiatrist, as extreme cases of demoralized inner worlds. The first of these threats is the threat of 'engulfment' by which is meant that the self feels itself in danger of being swallowed up by another self, resulting in its complete annulment and loss of identity. When the self feels itself to be in danger of being engulfed, it flees from people into isolation. As Laing points out, such a patient may well fear to be engulfed by his therapist. Therefore he resists the efforts of the doctor who tries to understand him. 'It is lonely and painful to be always misunderstood, but there is at least from this point of view a measure of safety in isolation [41]'.

The second menace to the security of a person's inner world is 'implosion', an obliteration of the self, a crashing in of his world which leaves only an empty shell. This anxiety, too, has an important effect on the treatment. The individual feels empty. 'Although in other ways he longs for the emptiness to be filled, he dreads the possibility of this happening because he has come to feel that all he can be is that awful nothingness of just this very vacuum. Any "contact" with reality is then in itself experienced as a dreadful threat because reality, as experienced from this position, is necessarily *implosive* and thus, as was related in engulfment, *in itself* a threat to what identity the individual is able to have [42]'.

Laing calls the third threatened extreme loss of selfhood 'petrification': 'a particular form of terror, whereby one is petrified, i.e. turned to stone, the dread of this happening ... the "magical" act whereby one may attempt to turn someone else into stone, by "petrifying" him'. This is 'the act whereby one negates the other person's autonomy, ignores his feelings, regards him as a thing, kills the life in him. In this sense one may perhaps better say that one depersonalizes him, or reifies him. One treats him not as a person, as a free agent, but as an it [43]'. The moral implications of 'petrification' are obvious. 'Implosion' and 'engulfment' can also implicate the other morally if they are carried out as deliberate acts against the threatened person. But often such deeds are done without one's being aware of what one is doing to another person. In all cases in which a personality is threatened, the existential therapist must try to prevent such destruction by making the people concerned aware of the effects of their deeds. It is, of course, very important for the therapist to appreciate the demoralized state of a patient and to be aware of the results this condition may have on his attitude towards the doctor.

The need for considering what is unconscious, in the patient or in the person who damages the patient's self, illustrates further the need for integrating the existential and phenomenological elements within a medical framework. The introduction of the concept of the unconscious raises a methodological problem, however, for in the Husserlian conception there are only 'data of consciousness' while in most existentialist views there is only the freedom of the conscious mind and of his conscious choice. The existential therapist cannot, however, disregard the revolution which Freud brought about by establishing the fact that conscious feelings and decisions often are the results of unconscious processes [44].

The existential psychiatrist, in his concern for the patient's conscience, requires clinical judgement in deciding:

(a) whether to make a patient who is unaware of the voice of his conscience aware of it, and

(b) whether to trust the patient's moral judgement.

For, in cases of mental illness, a patient's sense of right and wrong may be distorted. He may, therefore, disregard the voice of conscience which the patient hears. Even in such cases, however, he still tends to interpret the patient's symptoms, his experience within his world, in terms of a desire to be an authentic person, i.e. in ethical terms.

In addition to considering the voice of the patient's conscience as residing in the unconscious and to interpreting his symptoms as indicating an unconscious striving for authenticity, the existential therapist must be aware of certain unconscious processes which affect all human experience and which limit the individual's freedom.

The psycho-analyst assumes that the analysand has certain experiences of which he is not conscious, such as identification with his father or hatred for his mother. Confirmation of the assumption is found in such conscious experiences as the feeling of being drawn to the same values as his father or the hatred of women who are in some way similar to his mother. These unconscious experiences determine a person's attitudes and his inner world; they are irrational and are in his phantasy. Some of them originate from contact with other people, for experience can be shared. Therefore, R. D. Laing speaks of 'a social phantasy system [45]'. As an example he quotes the experience of the analyst Bion who experienced being manipulated by a group of patients. The reverse is, of course, also true; the patients are drawn into their therapist's experience. The existential therapist must be aware of such phenomena, as they are relevant with regard to his patient achieving authenticity. He may find that the members of the patient's family form a 'nexus' and through being in collusion with one another deprive the patient of his authenticity [46].

The social phantasy system plays an important part in existential psychiatry. People manipulate each other consciously and unconsciously, and thus deprive one another of their authenticity. The existential therapist must be aware of these relationships and make patients and those who have an influence on them conscious of their intentions and the effects of their attitude. Thus a person may be freed from the bondage of a social nexus.

Many unhappy marriages consist of such entanglements, the stronger partner having enslaved the weaker person. Both become inauthentic as a result. The weak personality in spite of its protests has as a rule asked to be taken over. Each of them lives in his or her world and is not aware of the other's experience. The existential therapist can help them to gain insight into their situation and can encourage them to establish a true selfhood in a true relationship.

The weak person is frightened of the responsibilities of life, but at the same time suffers from self-contempt because of the failure to shoulder these responsibilities. The marriage partner becomes a scapegoat, and endless quarrels result.

Apart from the disappointment which a person experiences at his own weakness, there is the disappointment often felt by women at their husband's weakness for which they cannot forgive him, as they cannot forgive themselves for having married a weak man. Some solve the problem through a divorce, others stay in the unhappy relationship as a duty to the husband or to the children which they have borne him. The existential therapist encounters a difficult task when he has to help a woman to become reconciled to such a marriage.

Apart from being caught in a phantasy system or in a life situation, people are held in bondage by emotions. The existential psychiatrist must be aware of this danger to his patient's freedom. Sartre has pointed out that our whole world is experienced according to our emotional state and that our emotions have a convincing effect, that we believe in the world as it is coloured by them. Thus the self finds itself enveloped in gloom or in happiness, or in some other feeling. Emotion is, in Sartre's words, 'a certain way of apprehending the world, it is a transformation of the world, an abrupt drop of consciousness into the magical [47]'.

The existential psychiatrist has to fit the existential-phenomenological approach into a medically-orientated framework. For this purpose, he must consider all the factors which are relevant for mental health. These are the genetic endowment, processes taking place in the brain, stimuli conveying emotions to the mind, the instinctual energy and its control by the mind's rational power, irrational forces which require integration and past and present social influences. Viewed from the phenomenological point of view, these factors become experiences and their deterministic character is perceived by the person concerned as fate; it may be felt as a handicap imposed by the constitution, such as a tendency to depression, as an acquired disability, for instance the aftermath of a stroke with its inability to think clearly and to perform normal muscular movements, as the incapacity resulting from emotional impressions during childhood, as the power of instinctual desire, as the experience of manhood or womanhood or as a pressure of the social milieu. Seen from the ethical point of view, such experiences become challenges. The therapist must weigh their power against the patient's moral strength.

The existential psychiatrist, concerned with ethical and phenomenological questions, does not primarily classify his patients according to the psychiatric categories of specific mental illnesses. He cannot, however, ignore such classification, as it enables him to arrive at some orientation and, in addition, characterizes the different worlds in which his patients live by reference to some form of diagnostic label. But in making this classification he must never fail to look for the ethical principle and must consider the patient's illness as the result of not having coped with the tasks of life. An account will now be given of some diseases of the mind, considered from the phenomenological-existential standpoint within a medical framework. The diagnostic label will be attached to the patient suffering from the particular disorder.

THE FRAMEWORK OF THE PSYCHIATRIC DIAGNOSIS

The Compulsive-Obsessional

The world of the compulsive-obsessional person is dominated by rituals which, he feels, must be carried out to appease fate or to prevent intolerable anxiety from overtaking him. The rituals which may involve thought processes or actions seem unintelligible at first, but further investigation may reveal an underlying conflict of which they are but the expression. Such a conflict may be interpreted as ethical. Two cases in Henderson and Gillespie's *Text Book of Psychiatry* [48] illustrate this point. The first case is that of a clergyman who 'had distressing impulses to sing "Dim-dam-dimnity" to the tune of some hymn'. The explanation given by Henderson and Gillespie is as follows: '. . . the obsession to use profane language symbolized his desire to be rid of the burdensome restrictions of his calling [49]'. The other case concerns a girl who 'had such a persistent obsessive fear of bichloride of mercury tablets that she remained confined to her room for two years'. Investigation revealed that 'she associated in her mind such tablets with an illicit pregnancy'; and the authors add: '. . . which she had both desired and feared [50]'. Both these patients were beset by a conflict which concerned vital questions of right and wrong. Their illness was an expression of their inability to face the conflict and to act in good conscience. Existential psychotherapy in such a case consists in bringing the conflict before the patient's conscious mind and in trying to help him to resolve the conflict.

The Depressive

A compulsive-obsessional patient lives in a bleak world, dominated by rituals, and therefore feels depressed. There are, however, others who live in a world of depression without ritualistic features. They experience life as monotonous, empty and without meaning. They live in the shadow of darkness and cannot see any light in the future. These people demonstrate the truth of Sartre's observations about the power of emotions: they are caught in a gloomy world where gloom is of their own constitution. They provide also an instance of a mental illness affecting conscience so that it ceases to be the reliable arbiter of right and wrong. The psychiatrist has to know that the self-accusations of the depressed patient, his professions of guilt with regard to himself and others have no moral basis, but are just manifestations of his illness. These feelings disappear when the patient has received successful treatment. Therefore these guilt feelings cannot form the basis of existential psychotherapy. Still, there are unmistakable signs of a moral struggle in the depressed person. In resisting the temptation to commit suicide, he shows moral courage, facing and enduring his painful life.

In certain cases of depression, there is a precipitating event such as a severe disappointment at being jilted, with which the person could not cope. To the existential therapist the state of depression has come about because of lack of moral strength. His task consists in helping the patient to cope, i.e. to live with the disappointment or just to face the state of depression as a burden. The use of physical measures such as electric convulsion treatment and drugs must always be considered, if the existential approach should fail.

The Manic

This ghastly world of depression can change miraculously for the patient. The opposite features can take the place of those characterizing depressions. The patient has swung into a manic phase. He is now overactive and full of optimism. He can, however, not carry out his intentions, as he cannot concentrate on what he is doing. He does not realize his limitations. Although the swing into a manic phrase may come about as part of a constitutional tidal wave, there are cases in which an unconscious moral factor plays a part which the existential psychiatrist can make the basis of his treatment. Henderson and Gillespie mention such a possibility in their text-book. The fictitious patient is an adult woman who had been tied to her father and had hated her mother without being conscious of this hatred (consciousness would have caused her guilt feelings, too deep to bear). When the mother died, her wish to get rid of her was fulfilled and she became manically elated. To her conscious mind the elation was causeless, yet she was completely in the power of this emotion [51]. To the existential psychotherapist this woman's 'guilt' lies in her failure to have grown up. The 'guilty' party would be the father if he had discouraged the daughter to lead an authentic life. These are the insights which the treatment would convey to the patient. The therapist has to assess the patient's ability to bear the emotional strain of accepting such interpretation: if she is unable to do so, drugs must be given which reduce her excitement and which may, of course, also make her capable of facing the moral problem.

The Schizophrenic

Let us first carry out a *phenomenological* analysis of schizophrenia. We find that the world of such a person is characterized by isolation. He lives enclosed in a system of ideas. He has lost touch with reality completely; he does not care about people or behaviour. He may feel anger and irritability or he may be quite indifferent and apathetic. His own body feels strange and dead, as does his whole personality. He may believe that people are against him and hear their hostile voices or imagine that they have set traps for him (paranoid schizophrenia). The self of the schizophrenic is empty and hollow. L. Binswanger has given a vivid description of how such a patient experiences the world and herself [52]. She described her own situation by saying: 'I feel myself excluded from all real life. I am quite isolated. I sit in a glass ball. I see people through a glass wall, their voices come to me muffled. I have an unutterable longing to get to them. I scream, but they do not hear me. I stretch out my arms toward them; but my hands merely beat against the walls of my glass ball [53]'. E. Minkowski has also given a revealing account of the world of one of his patients suffering from a schizo-phrenic depression [54]. This patient's experience of time is described as follows: 'Each day kept an unusual independence, failing to be immersed in the perception of any life continuity; each day life began anew, like a solitary island in a gray sea of passing time. What had been done, lived, and spoken no longer played the same roles as in our life because there seemed to be no wish to go further, every day was an exasperating monotony of the same words, the same complaints, until one felt that this being had lost all sense of necessary continuity. Such was the march of time for him.

'However, our picture is still incomplete; an essential element is missing in it — the fact that *the future was blocked* by the certainty of a terrifying and destructive event. This certainly dominated the patient's entire outlook and absolutely all of his energy was attached to this inevitable event [55]'. Another feature of this psychic state re-ported by Minkowski was that this man could not learn from his experience as normal people do. He was deluded and was awaiting his execution in a state of terror every night. The fact that it always failed to take place did not in the least comfort him. He could not generalize, drawing conclusions from the experience of safety in the past to being safe in the future.

The experience of time, space, materiality and of causality is greatly disturbed in the schizophrenic as the above accounts illustrate [56]. In the depressed schizophrenic, the space is dark, the body is empty, there is no awareness of causality and matter and substance take part to form the world of madness in which these people live.

The features revealed by the phenomenological analysis must now be viewed from the ethical, *existential* point of view. Such interpretation illustrates a number of points already made in the exposition of the general existential theory of mental illness. Campbell is quoted in Henderson and Gillespie's text-book as having come to the conclusion that the symptoms of this illness must be understood in moral terms, as 'a surrender, the challenge of life appearing too great [57]'. R. D. Laing even cites the story of one of his own schizophrenic patients whose conscience was raised into consciousness and who gained insight into her so far unconscious self-destruction as a result of a film in which she saw in the main character her own self, cut off from life. The heroine of the film, however, had not given up the struggle; inspired by the example, the patient ceased the destruction of her own identity [58].

So far as the aetiology of the disease is concerned, Laing has pointed out that many such patients, during their childhood, were denied the security of love and authentic relationship in which a child is confirmed in its value by the other members of the family [59]. Social psychiatry which is existentially-orientated considers these influences and tries to rehabilitate the patient's personality by respecting him as a member of the community [60].

The Hysteric

The hysteric cannot face life and withdraws into a world of phantasy and of pretence. He (or she) may be suffering from various bodily manifestations of the illness such as muscular weakness or loss of voice or from such mental disturbances as loss of memory or dream-like states. Again the patient is not conscious of the significance of the symptoms. In his book on emotion, Sartre cites an incident which illustrates the form of inauthenticity exhibited by such people and which shows how they become enmeshed in their own emotional network.

The case is that of a woman whose original intention had been to make a confession to her doctor, but such a confession was a task that was too painful for her. She therefore unconsciously abdicated her power to speak. She became hysterical and was 'shaken with tears and hiccoughs'. She also projected her difficulties on to the world which, she imagined, demanded that she should go through the agony of a confession. As Sartre points out, the difficulties of her situation were not faced and became impossible to face, as she had exaggerated them until they became to her unbearable. She now found herself in a world of gloom and sadness in which she had no freedom to communicate as a free self with others. Thus she was caught in a nexus of inauthenticity, sorrow and fear of the world towards which she felt hostility and from which she hid herself, having abandoned responsibility [61].

As the examples of the different diseases show, the existential-phenomenological approach can be integrated within a medical framework. We shall now examine the contributions made by medical psychologists from the existential point of view which will thus be further elucidated.

An Existential Re-Interpretation of Some Central Insights of Traditional Medical Psychologies

While schools of medical psychology recognize the significance of the unconscious in general — this being their major contribution — they have interpreted unconscious experience in terms of their particular naturalistic theories and have therefore done violence to the understanding of the ethical dimension of the patient. As the concerns of these schools are also vital concerns of the existential psychiatrists, they must be viewed from a new standpoint.

We shall examine the *Freudian* view first. According to its theory, neurotic symptoms result from the damming back of the instinctual flow, the patient's anxiety being explained as the result of the suppression of this energy, which the treatment then aims at releasing. By contrast, the existential viewpoint regards the sexual urge as a challenge with which the patient has to cope and which endangers the integrity of his personality. It is the recognition of this danger which causes anxiety according to the existentialist view. The difference in these interpretations can be illustrated by a concrete example.

Masturbation is for the Freudian just a way of gaining sexual pleasure and satisfaction and is abnormal only in so far as the expression by intercourse is thereby prevented. To the existential psychiatrist, however, the act is of potential danger to the self. Distinction must be made between masturbation which occurs during childhood and adolescence as part of the normal process of maturation, or in special circumstances when a love-partner is lacking, and masturbation which has become addiction, often being associated with such perversions as fetishism, exhibitionism and homosexuality, and which thereby threatens the integrity of the self. The juvenile form, which is part of the natural development, can become the self-damaging habit. Mutual masturbation must be included as part of this evaluation. The decisive question in determining the existence of mutual masturbation is whether the aim is purely physical pleasure or whether bodily stimulation and satisfaction are subordinated to a loving devotion to the partner [62].

The above distinction is concerned only with the actual damage to the self and therefore does not indicate any difference between the Freudian and the existential therapists regarding juvenile sexuality. There is, however, a very real difference: the psycho-analyst ignores the feeling of threat to the personality which is caused by the sexual urge, while the existential psychiatrist recognizes that sexual desire is experienced as an important aspect of the existential situation.

Although the existential psychiatrist differs radically in his views from the Freudian, he nonetheless acknowledges the contributions which Freud has made to the phenomenology of mental life. Freud's analysis of the occurrence of slips of the tongue, his accounts of the rising of emotions into the focus of consciousness, of the reliving of forgotten events in a state of relaxation, are all recognized by the existential psychiatrist to be contributions of great significance for the understanding of the inner worlds of human beings [63].

Jung, who rejected Freud's theory, accepted the ethical principle. This acceptance was, however, invalidated by the adoption of the naturalistic standpoint. It is Jung's naturalistic determinism which provides the fundamental ground of opposition between the Jungian and the existential psychiatrist. Both stress the moral character of the self; but to the Jungian, the self is an archetype and thus belongs to the impersonal collective unconscious, and not exclusively to the individual person to whom it only conveys an ideal. To the existentialist, the self is 'the always present existential ground of being [64] '.

Both the Jungian and existential approaches are concerned with fundamental experience: apart from selfhood there is manhood, womanhood, evil (in Jungian terms 'the shadow') and others. However, Jung sought in accordance with scientific method to derive these subjective elements from an objective principle. They are turned into archetypes which, we found, he defined as 'the a priori determining constituents of all experience', conceived as 'inherited psychic qualities [65] ', and located into a physical object, the brain structure.

As a result of the deterministic framework, into which the archetypes are introduced, they operate as a fate of a person against which he has little power. In the existential situation, on the other hand, experiences are primary, they *are* the 'data of consciousness' in the Husserlian sense. The self has the task of coping with them, they are challenges and the self's freedom to deal with them is not jeopardized by a theory: thus understood, Jung's psychology like that of Freud's conveys vital information to the existential psychiatrist.

In contrast to the Freudians and the Jungians, and in common with the existentialist, the *Adlerian* school accepts experience as something primary and understands a person from the point of view of his subjective striving, his 'style of life' which manifests his general aim and his goal. Within this orientation, Adler has made a valuable contribution to understanding people by drawing attention to the significance of the feeling of inferiority which arises when a person compares himself with others, and finding himself to be less good than they are. This situation is always found in childhood. The assessment depends on the standards which the person has set for himself. Feelings of inferiority are liable to occur when people are affected by physical and mental illnesses which interfere with their capacity to hold their own. They cause great suffering, leaving the person insecure and frightened of others. In the neurotic, such experience is very marked. The self has to find a way out. Adler showed great insight when he observed that the new goal is the attainment of power and superiority to compensate for the feeling of inferiority. If these aims are reached in practice, however, the person becomes unpopular with his fellow human beings and suffers loneliness because he is shunned. He may, of course, pursue such aims in phantasy, but he then loses touch with reality.

When Adler investigated the dynamics of subjective striving in this way, he contributed positively to the clarification of the existential situation. When, however, he imposed his concept of the 'social interest' on his patients' experience, he did violence to the existential situation and to the ethical principle. The following example illustrates how his theory led him to offend against the authenticity of a patient's self.

The case concerns a girl of eleven, afraid to go to school and in treatment by Adler. He wrote: 'On the mornings of the schooldays she is so nervous that the whole house suffers'. It is obvious that the girl was genuinely terrified of school and that she upset her family because of her terror. In order to confirm the theory of superiority and to vindicate the 'ethics of the social interest', Adler interpreted her behaviour as an unconscious effort to gain superiority over her family: 'she enjoys complete domination over her family, yet does not understand this fact in its context'. He went on to say: 'If she could be made to realize the truth, if we could show her that the extreme overrating of the varying problems of school is nothing but bragging and constructing an alibi for possible failure to excel at school, we should be taking an important step in the right direction. We may go further and show her what type of person brags. No one will try to impress other people unless he believes that his actual accomplishments give insufficient testimony of his personal importance'. Thus to the already present terror of school was added the feeling of guilt towards her family and shame on account of her poor performance in her lessons. This guilt served as a pressure on her to make her accept her doctor's views, to agree that she was spoilt and to say to herself when upset: 'Dr. Adler would say that I did that just to show off'. Adler, confident in his superiority over the child, viewed this development as inevitable: '... the time will come', he wrote, 'when in the very midst of the tumult, she will remember how her conduct would appear to me' and added: '... this self-consciousness alone will effect great improvement. And finally she will wake up in the morning with the realization: "Now I'm about to stir up a commotion in the family". And being aware of it, she can then avoid it [66]'.

Adler's patient was prevented from coming to terms with her existential situation, from facing the real problem which school presented to her. She was not given a chance to understand herself because of the application of a schematic theory. She was not regarded by her doctor as a free being and therefore was not allowed to make a decision which might be called her own. The case shows the effect which the adoption of Vaihinger's relativistic philosophy of the as-if had on Adler's psychotherapy: the reduction of the ethical principle to a useful fiction and damage caused as a result to the self of the patient [67].

The Patient's Struggle for Faith

The patient has to come to terms with his instinctual urges, his 'archetypal' experiences, his feelings of inferiority and his longing for power and for superiority. He has to face the challenges with which these experiences present him. In his struggle the patient stands in need of a *faith* which will sustain him. This faith must be in something absolute, transcendental, in something which is independent of the vicissitudes of changing experiences. Although such a principle cannot be known, it can be experienced.

One way in which the patient is in danger of losing the struggle for faith is through the modern tendency to make the particular despair which has come about through the 'death' of God into a universal and inevitable fate. This tendency to universalize particular experiences is an attribute of the human mind which desires to find in *one* principle the explanation of everything. This attribute is the metaphysical desire.

Certain existential philosophers have been referred to as the authors of ontologies, but their claim of having found the basis of human existence was rejected on epistemological and ethical grounds. It was admitted, however, that such existential ontologies have truth value for the people who find in them correct descriptions of the world in which they live. If the existential ontology describes a sick and hopeless world, however, the psychiatrist must regard such a view as dangerous to a person's faith and health.

Sartre and Heidegger are the authors of ontologies which depict the dilemma of modern man; he can see his image in their works, a being suffering from anxiety and in despair. Both these philosophies have been claimed as a suitable basis for the treatment of mentally ill people. Patients are harmed, however, if they accept such ontologies in their struggle for faith because they leave no room for faith.

The Ontologies of Sartre and Heidegger

SARTRE'S ONTOLOGIES

Many Sartrian characters are sick and show symptoms like those quoted earlier in the section on the phenomenology of the false self. These characters have been constructed to illustrate the consequence arising from the acceptance (to Sartre the inevitable acceptance) of a certain ontology.

Roquentin, the hero of Sartre's early novel *Nausea* suffers from feelings of nausea, not as something accidental, but as an expression of human existence as such. Although fully accepting the need for action, action appears to be useless. His sickness is 'profound boredom', which he calls 'the profound heart of existence', of which he says that it is '... the very matter I am made of [68]'. He feels out of touch with things and with people around him. He envies the way they feel at home in life and confident. They look forward to a future which is a natural continuation of their past. Roquentin cannot experience such continuity. The objects of the world, such as the root of a tree, confront him with the very question of why they exist at all. He cannot answer this question. Therefore, he argues, existence is absurd. In this insight, according to Sartre, Roquentin 'found the key to Existence', to his Nausea, to his whole life: absurdity is 'fundamental [69]'.

This novel throws light on a basic problem with which people are faced and which contributes to their state of insecurity greatly, thus making them liable to break down. Roquentin is right, there is no intelligible order of things in this world, the world is therefore absurd. A person's life shares in this arbitrariness, in this absurdity. Through his character, Sartre formulates this situation in the following way: 'I am free: there is absolutely no more reason for living, all the ones I have tried have given way and I can't imagine any more of them . . . My past is dead . . . I am alone in this white, garden-rimmed street. Alone and free. But this freedom is rather like death [70]'.

Although there is this absurdity, Sartre is wrong that man cannot

MEDICINE AND ETHICS   147

live with it. The fact that life is characterized by contingency does not in itself mean that there is no reason for living. Patients who feel and argue like Roquentin can be shown that life has its value even if there is no universal order, that man can have faith.

Sartre's *Being and Nothingness* [71] provides further insight into the effects which the belief in a particular ontology can have upon the mental health of the person who holds such belief. The relationship between one man and another, as conceived in this work by Sartre, has become more pathological than in his earlier *Nausea*: 'While I attempt to free myself from the hold of the Other, the Other is trying to free himself from mine; while I seek to enslave the Other, the Other seeks to enslave me [72]'. The psychiatrist calls such a view sadistic, masochistic and paranoid.

The ontological basis of this state of affairs is the assumption that my subjectivity, my freedom, is my consciousness; by becoming the object of another's consciousness – by being just looked at by him – my freedom, i.e. my authenticity or my selfhood, is destroyed. If I try to become the object of the Other's consciousness, I seek the destruction of my own freedom, the escape from my responsibilities. If I try to become conscious of myself, I have made myself into an object and have destroyed my own freedom. If I become conscious of the Other, it is only to make him *my* object. Thus the Sartrian ontology asserts the inevitableness of mutual and self-destruction. The insolubility of the dilemma of freedom is deduced from a fundamental ontology which calls freedom 'being for itself' and at the same time makes it dependent on 'being-in-itself' which is a thing without freedom: 'the for-itself without the in-itself is a kind of abstraction; it could not exist any more than a color could exist without form or a sound without pitch and without timbre [73]'. Freedom is, however, the essence of faith.

Anxiety is part of human life, but the Sartrian man is in a *continuous* state of anguish as a result of this postulated ontology. He has no true selfhood and does not feel that his life is justified or justifiable. 'In anguish we do not simply apprehend the fact that the possibles which we project are perpetually eaten away by our-freedom-to-come, in addition we apprehend our choice – i.e. ourselves – as *unjustifiable* [74]'.

The Sartrian man stands apart and watches himself acting, pretending. He is aware of his insincerity, his 'bad faith'. The Sartrian waiter goes through the movements of being a waiter, but lacks the conviction of being a person in this profession; the same applies to so many other characters met in Sartrian novels and plays. Psychiatrists can recognize the phenomenology of their schizoid and hysterical patients in these characters. Sartre has asked that his views should form the basis of the so-called 'existential psycho-analysis', but they are not suitable for treating mentally sick people because of their pessimistic nature.

HEIDEGGER'S ONTOLOGY

Whereas the Sartrian ontologies have not been officially adopted as a basis for psychiatry, a group of existential psychiatrists on the Continent have accepted Martin Heidegger's ontology as the foundation of their treatment. His views differ somewhat from Sartre's.

What is man's existence like if we accept Heidegger's scheme of things? We find a lonely person like Sartre's man. Care, i.e. anxious concern, forms the basis of his existence. He feels solicitous towards others. Although he admits that he lives in a world with them, they become his enemies when he tries to be authentic; for they are the crowd, given to 'idle talk', to 'curiosity', to 'ambiguity' which leads to 'the downward plunge' involving 'temptation, tranquillizing, alienation and self-entangling [75]'.

One cannot deny that Heidegger's phenomenological description of the mentality of the crowd and its danger to the individual who attempts to reach authenticity are true. The objection to this philosophy lies in its claim that this particular form of human existence is the only way to exist and that it is unalterable.

To the psychiatrist M. Boss, Heidegger's system is the basis of 'a new phenomenological science of man [76]'. What Boss expects of such a science is something which no science can provide: 'it ought to give us a thoroughly grounded understanding of the nature of such a personality-concept [of a personality which accepts responsibility and freedom], along with information as to whom a person really has to be responsible and why. Finally, it should give us insight into the nature of human freedom from what and for what a man should be free, and in what human freedom actually consists [77]'. The serious mistake in this exposition is the inclusion of ethics within science and the expectation that any science can provide an account of the nature of man. Heidegger's analysis of human existence is for Boss fundamental. According to him the 'psychiatric analysis of human existence' is to derive its elements from it, it is interpreted as a 'regional ontology', a section of the 'fundamental ontology [78]'. These statements point to the fact that Boss' patients are (consciously or unconsciously) led to experience their existence in terms of Heidegger's ontology. This amounts to a serious interference with their freedom and to a distortion of their world of experience [79].

NON-ONTOLOGICAL POSITIVE EXISTENTIAL PHILOSOPHIES

Kierkegaard offers the psychiatrist a starting point for his endeavour of treating the patient who is in despair over his situation and who is struggling for faith; for Kierkegaard realized that despair was the 'passage-way to faith [80]'. Kierkegaard also recognized that we cannot expect faith to be easily won. Before we can 'make the great leap', we may have to go through a stage of resignation when faith is absent. The movement of faith 'must constantly be made by virtue of the absurd [81]'. Thus faith emerges as a miracle, a manifestation of strength which a man finds after a period of despair. The doctor has to stand by during the time of resignation; he must be aware of the moment when his patient gathers the strength for the leap and he can rejoice with him in his triumph over the absurd. In order to prepare the ground for this movement of faith, the psychiatrist must understand the situation of absurdity which gave rise to the despair in the first place. Roquentin found life absurd because of its arbitrariness, its incongruity and the absence of any intelligible order. It is this sort of experience which gives rise to many nervous breakdowns, as indeed was the case with Roquentin.

There are several answers; one of them is: although men cannot see any order in life, such order may exist beyond the level of human intelligence. Congruity is a demand made by human reason; religion relies on faith which, as Kierkegaard pointed out, proves itself by the acceptance of the absurd [82].

Modern western man lives consciously in a rational world of science and technology. Many strive from within this world for faith in God. The doctor must be aware of the patient's conflict and may have to co-operate with a priest making intelligible the existential situation of 'credo quia absurdum est'. He must, however, leave the main task of helping him in this struggle to the minister of religion.

To those who do not find the solution of the riddle of life in God, there is no conception which could explain the inconsistencies and the meaning of life as a whole. Man is faced with ultimate absurdity; how then can he gain faith in a transcendental principle? The second answer to the dilemma is that he has to find faith manifested in himself, in experiences which confirm the transcendental nature of his selfhood. Camus has shown in his book *The Myth of Sisyphus* [83] how man can avoid despair and can have faith in himself in face of the absurd.

Sisyphus' fate is symbolic of the existential situation of a person who has to toil without respite and who does not achieve a satisfactory result at the end. He is all alone. His labour is fruitless and monotonous. According to the myth, Sisyphus was condemned by the Gods to roll a stone up a mountain without ever reaching the top; the stone would always roll down before his effort was successful, and then his labour would begin again. For Sisyphus, therefore, there is no future to look forward. There is only the present, the pressing task of lifting the stone another inch or going down the mountain to resume the senseless task. Such a man, faced with such absurdity, can avoid despair by being resigned to the fact that there is no future. There is only the present. 'Sisyphus teaches the higher fidelity that negates the Gods and raises rocks ... This universe without a master seems to him neither sterile nor futile. Each atom of that stone, each mineral flake of that night-filled mountain, in itself forms a world. The struggle itself towards the heights is enough to fill a man's heart. One must imagine Sisyphus happy [84] '.

Camus further developed the theme of the lonely man faced with a hopeless task in the novel *The Plague* [85]. The hero is Dr Rieux who carries on a fight against the plague with insufficient means. The suffering of humanity is absurd to him and he refuses to accept the priest's suggestion: 'Perhaps we should love what we cannot understand'. His answer is: 'Until my dying day I shall refuse to love a scheme of things in which children are put to torture [86] '. Dr Rieux is sustained in his work by his responsibility as a doctor, which he defined as a 'struggle with all our might against death [87] '. He is a resolute man insisting that all possible steps against the plague should be taken when others were afraid to face the danger. He acts as a man who is not afraid to stand apart from the crowd, makes his decisions and is not paralyzed by the absurd. In *The Plague* Camus has put forward a view shared by Jaspers that a man who is in danger of foundering in despair can save himself by discovering the transcendental in himself and can achieve confirmation of his selfhood in the moment of choice and decision. In resolution he gains his faith.

The psychiatrist who wants to apply these insights to the existential situations met in his practice must be aware of the fact that his patients are severely handicapped in their freedom to make decisions and choices. We have seen how they are hemmed in: the compulsive-obsessional having to perform his rituals, the depressive living in a world of darkness in which every thought and movement is slowed down, the manic unable to concentrate, the schizophrenic enclosed in a system of phantasy experiencing his future blocked and the hysteric living a life of pretence having detached himself from his actions. Although the neurotic is freer than the psychotic, he finds a decision terrifying, as it means giving up one thing in favour of another. He feels so insecure that he wants to hold on to everything. The psychiatrist who has recognized his patient's weakness must wait patiently before sufficient strength for even a small leap is available. Then he must encourage the sick man to dare to make the leap, and to find his true ground. Existential psychotherapy involves the liberation of what Jaspers calls 'philosophical faith' which is 'the fundamental source of that work by which man makes himself in an inner act as an individual before his Transcendence [88]'.

The therapist must remember that the patient's concern for convention and for the approval of others constitutes a great obstacle to gaining selfhood through personal decision. Jaspers is emphatic in castigating irresolution as a compromise which is not made in the interest of others but out of cowardice, and which thus reveals a lack of selfhood. He encourages men to face their alternatives: 'When, in any matter, a man is wholly himself, he recognizes that there are alternatives, and then his action will not be a compromise [89]'. It is the task of the therapist to disclose to the patient the authenticity he seeks and the consequent need for decision which he must take.

Philosophical faith in Jaspers' sense, however, is not exhausted by the act of decision. Indeed, philosophical faith 'is inseparable from complete openness to communication and 'the will to boundless communication . . . is the very essence of philosophical faith [90]'. By communication Jaspers means joining the world of another man; this communication is existentially imperative for 'the only reality with which man can reliably and in self-understanding ally himself in the world, is his fellow man [91]. Through the bond between self and self the feeling of absurdity is overcome and the meaning of life is no more in question. The existential psychiatrist has to be aware of the possibility of communication and its power.

By affirming faith in the relation between man and man, Jaspers, in common with certain other existential philosophers, differs profoundly from Sartre and Heidegger, whose ontologies have been criticized for viewing 'the other' essentially as an enemy, and whose worlds are devoid of communication. Sartrian and Heideggerian men are lonely and many of Sartre's fictional characters, as was pointed out earlier on, exhibit the symptoms of mental patients.

The possibility of gaining faith through communication is of considerable importance in the patient's existential situation. As Martin Buber has written, the dialogical relation means 'being chosen and choosing [92]'; authentic dialogue occurs between whole people and has, as Buber says, a liberating effect. In the dialogical relation, both are enabled to gain faith in themselves and in each other. Their relationship is pure mutuality. This mutuality cannot last, however, and the one will become an object for the other. Then the faith between them is liable to be shaken. A patient must have the strength to live through this phase, when mutuality may be lost, and must then re-establish communication which can never be something taken for granted.

The question arises, however, whether those people who suffer from mental illness can enter into communication. Is this relationship not reserved for whole people, i.e. for those who have a capacity for wholeness in the Buberian sense? The answer is that just as the patient is handicapped with regard to his ability to make decisions, so must doubt arise concerning his ability to 'meet' the other. Is he then capable of gaining faith through relationships at all?

Jaspers and Buber appear to exclude many normal people, even from the possibilities of establishing communication. Jaspers says: 'Only he who is himself and can prove himself in solitude can truly enter into communication [93]'. And Buber remarks in reply to Heidegger: 'A genuine and adequate self . . . makes self be bound to self . . . it founds the communion of individuals [94]'. A psychiatric patient is certainly not 'one who has proved himself in solitude', he is not 'himself' and his self is not 'genuine' and 'adequate', or he would not be a patient. It is precisely because his self is false, a self in phantasy, that he has sought psychiatric aid. Indeed, it is the very lack of selfhood which characterizes the neurotic and the psychotic patient. They are, therefore, prevented from a dialogical relationship with others and are reduced to a monological relationship with themselves. In Buber's words 'Thou . . . strikes inwards. It develops on the unnatural, impossible object of the I, that is, it develops where there is no place at all for it to develop. Thus confrontation of what is over against him takes place within himself, and this cannot be relation, or presence, or streaming interaction, but only self-contradiction . . . Here is the verge of life, flight of an unfulfilled life to the senseless semblance of fulfilment, and its groping in a maze and losing itself ever more profoundly [95]'.

For the patient, then, dialogue and communication in the Buberian and Jasperian senses is impossible. These conceptions remain ideals to be striven for, but only rarely — and certainly not for the neurotic or psychotic person – achieved. On the other hand dialogue and communication, the establishment of relation, even in a modified way, are the means by which the sick person can gain a form of authenticity.

The existential psychiatrist must seek to help his patient who is caught in a phantasy system and whose situation is desperate primarily because he cannot reach his fellow men and, as a result, is beset by loss of faith. To aid him the therapist must establish that communication from which a restorative faith can spring.

In his endeavour to help the patient to leave his phantasy world, the existential therapist can rely on the patients' wish to reach the Other. Like Ellen West [96] people want to communicate with their fellow human beings. In trying to help the sick person to gain faith through communication with the Other, the therapist finds himself in the company of those theologians who try to help people who have lost their faith in the traditional teachings of the church but who are seeking to find 'a gracious God' in 'a gracious neighbour [97]'.

The therapist in his own efforts to help people to gain faith can find inspiration from Martin Buber. In his *I and Thou* Jewish, Christian and Buddhist teachings merge, and the human other is seen as the bearer of the divine eternal Thou, a Thou which unlike other 'thous' does not become an object. The faith which is of such vital importance for people who are isolated and lost in their existential vacuum, is the faith which emerges in human relationships, when they are truly dialogical and mutual: 'He who loves a woman and brings her life to present realisation in his, is able to look in the *Thou* of her eyes into the beam of the eternal Thou [98]'.

Communion with the other is the very basis on which human order is built and from which the sustaining faith of this order arises. For this reason the deliberate and conscious disregard of inter-human relations can only be regarded as *existential guilt*: 'Existential guilt occurs when someone injures an order of the human world whose foundations he knows and recognizes as those of his own existence and of all common human existence [99]'.

While guilt feelings may indicate the presence of existential guilt, psychiatrists must make allowance for the possibility that such feelings are deceptive. The guilt feelings of a depressed patient, for instance, were earlier described as symptoms of his disease and not related to any wrong thought or action. In the manic patient, considered above, feelings of guilt were interpreted as being the result of suppressed hatred, which the patient had not been able to face and for which she was therefore not responsible (the existential guilt might have to be attributed to the father if he had prevented his daughter from leading an authentic life). In the case of the schizophrenic, it was demonstrated that the patient himself did not bear the guilt, but those who had caused his withdrawal from society and were therefore responsible for his condition.

On the other hand, as a person endowed with conscience, a patient is capable of recognizing his existential guilt when he has, in fact, injured the inter-human order. The existential psychiatrist has a duty to help him to become aware of his own fundamental ability to believe in a moral human order. For his ability to believe in such an order can render his life meaningful [100].

There is the extreme case of the psychopathic personality, which is totally incapable of experiencing its obligations towards others and towards itself. The psychopath does not feel ill; he is resolute and shows his power of making decisions, often by anti-social behaviour. He does not appear, therefore, to be struggling towards any faith in humanity, and in so far as he is without conscience, is outside the reach of the existential approach.

Some psychopaths show, however, that they have at least unconsciously accepted the principle of the inter-human order; for they protest against the violation of this order in their own individual cases. They are filled with strong resentment against society which they blame for the lack of love they experienced earlier in their lives, especially during childhood. Such patients may be treated with existential psychotherapy and may have their faith in the value of human relations rekindled.

THE PSYCHOTHERAPEUTIC ENCOUNTER

The psychopath who is full of resentment against society meets the therapist with suspicion. The same is true of the patient who suffers from paranoia. Although, in general, neurotic and psychotic patients basically wish to make relations with their doctors, the psychiatrist must realize that they may be afraid of such relations, which may be experienced as threats to their own security. Laing's observations on 'engulfment', 'implosion' and 'petrification' should be recalled in this context. Patients may be intensely afraid of leaving their own world – no matter how uncomfortable it may be – for a new and untried world. 'The neurotic [and psychotic] takes fright when confronted with a change of his personality as if it were his death. Even at the cost of severe suffering he holds on to the fiction of an alleged security and constancy although he feels in the depth of his being that these are unreal . . . When this inflexibility begins to yield in the course of the treatment, the experience is that of having met his death [101] '. These words do not apply to all psychiatric patients but they give a true account of the paradox which Kierkegaard has described in his *The Sickness unto Death* [102] : 'A despairing man wants despairingly to be himself. But if he despairingly wants to be himself, he will not want to get rid of himself [103]'; for the present self, sick as it is, is the only self he possesses and this self would have to die in order to make room for a new healthier self to be born. In the therapeutic encounter the existential therapist has to give such a person the strength to go through this metamorphosis.

As the patient's self is sick, the patient cannot be expected to exist in the relationship with the doctor as an equal. This has been recognized and emphasized with great clarity by Martin Buber: 'In order that [the therapist] may coherently further the liberation and actualization of that unity [the unity of the suffering soul] in a new accord of the person with the world, the psychotherapist, like the educator, must stand again and again, not merely at his own pole in the bipolar relation, but also with the strength of present realization at the other pole, and experience the effect of his own actions [104]'.

The doctor must offer a love which differs from all other forms of love; it must be indestructible and available for all patients equally. Furthermore, the therapist must be aware of the patient's wish to make him a person in authority, to identify himself with the therapist and to accept his values unquestionably. He must be on guard against these tendencies [105].

The therapist must also possess and display a general understanding of the sick person in the psychotherapeutic encounter, an understanding which rests on his ability to reproduce the patient's world in his own world, and to 're-live' the patient's life, and to re-create his world. This understanding, which is the essence of the phenomenological approach, is identical with Dilthey's intuitive immediate understanding, which he distinguished from discursive, conceptual knowledge, characteristic of science [106].

Karl Jaspers, who had been a pupil of Dilthey, adapted Dilthey's approach for the psychotherapist. He developed an 'understanding psychology' and emphasized the fact that, in contrast to scientific knowledge, in his approach there is an immediate grasping of the origins of mental happenings, but no possibility of checking them through other observers. What 'proof' there is lies in intuition or empathy, and the method does not lead to discovery of causes or to universally valid propositions. The position in 'understanding psychology' is thus different from an objective understanding of the mind which, we found, was restricted to the organic approach which considers mental phenomena as manifestations of processes occurring in the brain.

An especially clear instance of the fallacy of drawing objectively valid general conclusions from the subjective experience of one particular person, is seen in the paper by a 'practising psychiatrist', entitled 'The Experience of Electro-Convulsive Therapy' and published in the *British Journal of Psychiatry* [107]. Although many patients to whom electro-convulsive treatment has been given, have declared that they found this experience terrifying, the author of this paper ignores their statements and, as he himself did not experience any terror, sets out to 'dispel the erroneous belief that this is a terrifying form of treatment'. He maintains that he can describe 'his subjective experience in objective terms' which, he implies, possess universal validity.

While 'understanding psychology' does not lead to propositions which possess universal validity, it does lead to descriptions which are dynamic and illuminating: 'Psychic events "emerge" out of each other in a way which we understand. Attacked people become angry and spring to the defence, cheated people grow suspicious. The way in which such emergence takes place is understood by us, our *understanding is genetic*. Thus we understand psychic reactions to experience, we understand the development of passion, the growth of an error, the content of delusion and dream; we understand the effects of suggestion, an abnormal personality in its context or the inner necessities of someone's life. Finally, we understand how the patient sees himself and how this mode of self-understanding becomes a factor in his psychic development [108]'.

The therapist who has understood the patient in his world communicates this picture to him, holding up a 'mirror' and reflecting a clarifying image, as it were, of his situation. Having gained insight into the elements of an actual set of circumstances in his life, the patient can begin to appreciate his potentialities in general, whether they are instinctual, intellectual, aesthetic, etc. [109]. Nowhere does the personal factor in the healing process reveal itself more positively than in those cases in which the therapist is successful in inspiring the patient with faith in those forces which are the bearers of his life [110]'.

The therapeutic encounter, however, must achieve more than merely providing the patient with insight into his situation and into the nature of the different functions of his psyche. It must help him to see what has caused his self to be in bondage and what keeps it in that state.

The source of psychiatric illness often lies in childhood. In the therapeutic encounter, submerged feelings of resentment are revived which emerged originally in experiences suffered at the hands of adults who had power over the patient when he was a child. People tend to generalize and to draw unwarrantable conclusions from such intense experiences and, as a result, adopt a hostile attitude towards the whole world [111]. The therapist has to be aware of this tendency and of the danger which it poses for the success of the treatment.

We have already seen that people who cannot enter into relations with others withdraw into a world of phantasy and become trapped in their phantasy system, which may take the form of a false paradise or of the hell of their early life. In the latter case, they are liable to repeat endlessly the painful situations of the past, perpetuating their suffering and their resentment.

The existential therapist who tries to free the patient from his unhealthy state of introversion must also be aware of a danger already mentioned: the acceptance by the patient of an ontology of despair. This ontological attitude typified by the Sartre of *Being and Nothingness* is attractive to these people who are already isolated; they accept this sort of *Weltanschauung,* which then envelops them emotionally and makes their world even more lonely. In order to counteract the compelling power of such an outlook, the therapist, in his encounter with the patient, must expose the fallacy of the ontological argument which supports it. This does not mean that he should engage his patients in philosophical discussions, it will not suffice to expose the fallacy of the argument logically. The fallacy of the argument has to be *experienced,* even as its 'truth' has already been experienced by the patient in his life. The feeling of overwhelming necessity ruling his existence must be dispersed. The patient must be infused with hope, with the recognition that his world need not be so bleak and lonely; his faith in the possibility of a world, different from what he has experienced, has to be awakened.

Existential psychotherapy involves discussing ultimate issues (life, death, meaning), but such discussion is not concerned with abstract philosophical reasoning. It is always concerned with the question of how a person is to orientate himself in a concrete situation, to make his life meaningful under the particular conditions of his life and to cope with its trials and conflicts.

Existential psychotherapy consists not only in making a patient aware of his situation, but also in standing by him while he is struggling to master it. Months or years may be required before he has achieved some degree of freedom which would allow him to cope with the problems gripping him.

There are no specific techniques for this form of treatment. The therapist who has adopted an existential ethics will find ways of applying techniques which are used by other psychological schools, adapting them for his purpose.

The patient may be treated in individual sessions, in groups or in a Therapeutic Social Club. In groups sometimes the plight of another patient helps him to see his own situation more clearly. He can experience confirmation of his selfhood in communication with the members of the group or club and not only with his therapist. He can learn to share his therapist with other patients.

The presence of others generally helps the patient to find a place in a community. He is given a chance to relate to them whether he visits a Social Therapeutic Club or takes part in group sessions. Both of these can be conducted on existential lines. For instance, one patient's dream may be discussed and interpreted as that person's existential problem. The other members of the group can then use the material of the dream as a means of gaining insight into their own problems. For instance, the dream may portray a person's dependence on his mother from which he is trying to free himself. Some other patients may have the same problem and some may have made more progress in their liberation than others. Such a discussion can have great value with people 'entering' into their own and into each other's worlds.

Living and working in a community helps also by bringing the patients face to face with the ordinary tasks of life: getting meals ready, handling materials in the workshop or even putting chairs into a circle. To a highly disturbed person, who lives in a world of insanity, such activities are of great significance.

Free association technique and dream analysis can also help a patient, as can inducing a state of relaxation or a hypnotic state. This is done, not in order to prepare a patient to receive the doctor's suggestions, but to allow him to see more clearly what he is doing with his life and what he ought to be doing with it. In the hypnotic or hypnoidal state, it may be helpful to suggest to the patient that he is imagining sitting in a theatre and looking at the stage (so called 'reverie technique'). Many people can play out the drama of their life in imagination and then apply the insight which they have gained in actual life situations. Another technique which enables a patient to see his problem more clearly is to paint whatever comes into his mind. Such pictures are often symbolic and must be interpreted if he is to see their significance. The interpretation can come from the patient himself, from members of a group   therapeutic club and from the therapist.

The showing of so-called Mental Health Films in a Therapeutic Club may also be helpful. They depict the crises and conflicts of patients.

The mere provision of experiences is never the aim of this treatment, as in fact the patient can become a slave to experiences which can be a means of evading the responsibilities of life. The goal, whatever the technique used, is to enable the patient to leave his world of falsehood and to establish himself as a more authentic person. By discussing the material which is obtained in such sessions, the therapist can convey to the patient where his potentialities in life lie, for people express in phantasy what moves them, even if they cannot realize these aims in actual life [112].

In the encounter with the therapist the patient is made aware of his struggle for freedom and for authenticity. He learns to recognize the strength and nature of the forces which have held him back, keeping his past alive, and which are preventing him now from achieving better health. In this battle for freedom the doctor is the person on whom the patient tests his strength and his faith in humanity as well. The question in the patient's mind is whether he will meet the same rejection and experience the same domination with the doctor as he did with his parents before.

The encounter is more than a 'transference' in the psycho-analytic sense. There is not just a repetition of feelings towards the people who have played a part in the person's past life, but new experiences arise through having entered into a new personal relation with the therapist. The aim is not only to make conscious emotional patterns but to liberate potentialities, especially in human communication.

Doctor and patient may have to cover the same ground again and again when they meet; for new attitudes cannot be gained quickly and the mind persists in its old habits. The doctor must have the necessary patience to allow his patient to change gradually. Insight into the patient's way of experiencing life can enable the therapist to play his part and not to expect quick results.

Apart from meeting with patients, the existential therapist seeks meetings with the people who are involved in the patient's life. He tries to provide all concerned with better understanding of the situation in which they are together, recognizing the fact that experience is shared. In extending his treatment to people who are in contact with the patient, the existential therapist differs from the Freudian who restricts interviews to the patient, as he is of the opinion that otherwise his own relationship with the patient would suffer.

The Experience of the Body

Existential psychotherapy has, so far, been viewed as a method for the treatment of neurotic or psychotic patients, i.e. for the treatment of the mind. Such an interpretation is too narrow, however, bodily experience also must be integrated within the world of experience as a whole, just as emotions of joy, anger, grief and resentment mean nothing unless they are conceived within the framework of the whole personality.

The preoccupation with physical phenomena as such, seen in isolation from the perceiving mind, has led to a neglect of the question of their significance to human beings. Doctors are trained to treat their patients' bodies as if they were inanimate objects. True, pain is avoided to a very large extent through the use of anaesthetics and analgesics. Moreover, the good intuitive doctor follows the existential-phenomenological approach, however, unconsciously, and takes into account the moral challenge of his patients' physical illness. He is aware, for example, of the patients' need for courage in facing operations and chronic or fatal diseases. On the other hand, many physicians and surgeons fail to meet their responsibilities in this regard. To numerous gynaecologists the patient's womb is just the organ to bear children. Such surgeons often expect a patient to agree readily to its removal after she has passed child-bearing age. To her, however, this organ is the essence of womanhood; therefore, to part with it is a terrible loss. This loss may have to be borne, but the doctor must be aware of the trial which his patient is facing and for which she needs his help. Whatever the illness may be, whether skin blemishes, varicose veins, short-sightedness or any other condition which changes the appearance of the body, such a condition requires an adjustment, acceptance or resignation, on the part of the patient, demanding moral courage and strength. If the doctor is to provide help, he must comprehend what is going on in the patient's world of experience.

The artificial separation of body and mind follows from Cartesian dualism, from the postulation of a realm of physical structures and another of consciousness. 'Only from this Cartesian viewpoint is it possible to speak of "the body alone". Such a view, however, is an explicitation that does not take into consideration the mode in which my body is given to me — namely, as "mine". . . . The body is *my* body in its participation in the conscious *self*. . . . *My* body, however, is *mine* through its mysterious reference to *me*, to the conscious *self* with which it has fused [113]'.

Experience of the body can be investigated from a neurological and from a psychological point of view. The former is concerned with the part played by the sensory organs and nerves which carry impulses to the brain: disturbances affect the body image which is, for instance, enlarged in cerebellar disease. The latter view studies the mechanisms by which the mind projects its ideas and energy into the body: patients feel physically strong or weak largely according to their emotional states; depersonalization, a frightening experience which occurs in a number of emotional disturbances, is characterized by lightness, heaviness, deadness of the body, or some of its parts, or by peculiar feelings which patients cannot describe although they experience them most vividly.

Some disturbances of body experience are associated with certain mental illnesses; hypochondriasis is particularly rich in such symptoms. As P. Schilder has pointed out, there is a tendency of the organ which manifests the hypochondriasis to become isolated from the rest of the body-image and to give the experience of a foreign body [114]. A paranoid patient may project his faeces into the outside world as prosecutors [115], a depressed person might feel deadness in the body as an expression of the deadness of the mind. Sexual excitement not only affects the sexual organs, but may be projected into any other part where the patient may not recognize its true nature.

Schilder has rightly pointed out that Gestalt psychologists have overstressed the static configuration in the preceptions of bodies, including the body-image [116]. The dynamic view, the fluidity of the image has thus been neglected. In fact, the image is never static, it changes with new associations, with a change in memory, will, tendencies and intentions [117].

A person's image of himself does not only depend upon physiological and psychological factors. The social milieu plays an important part. A person is sensitive to other persons' ideas and expectations. He dresses and carries himself to please them, to be approved by them. A disfiguring disease is not only hard to bear because of its effect on the bearer but especially on account of its anticipated effects on other people.

The physician can do more than support his patients' bearing of their bodily experiences. He can lead them towards greater awareness of the body and by so doing train them to attain better mental health. Such a training is in line with the existential-phenomenological approach, as it opens up new potentials for the growth of the personality.

J. H. Schultz is the author of one system of training which combines concentration with relaxation [118]. The patient relaxes and suggests to himself general calmness, heaviness and warmth of body, calmness of heart-beat, of respiration, warmth radiating from the nerves in the abdomen affecting the abdominal organs and coolness of his forehead. Through such exercises, carried out under the supervision of a specially trained doctor, the strain of modern life can be lessened and certain functional abnormalities, affecting various organs, can be successfully treated. Apart from the general calming effect, the patient finds his inner world enriched by the new experiences which are individual in character; he sinks into himself and achieves a state in which he can meditate. The training is related to Yoga practices, but is itself not based on any form of religion. Some of the patients, however, go beyond the mere psycho-physical plane. They achieve a state of contemplation on the basis of the calmness of mind combined with bodily awareness and relaxation. This advanced stage of the training is concerned with existential values, with the meaning of life.

From the phenomenological-existential point of view, there is, therefore, no such thing as purely bodily illness, there are only (mental) experiences of bodily states from which the patient suffers and which are liable to cause him anxiety. All these states require courage in facing them, and the doctor in whose care the patient is must be aware of the significance of the illness for the patient and for his moral struggle and provide the greatest possible help to the sufferer.

MEDICINE BASED ON EXISTENTIAL ETHICS

The existential-phenomenological approach and the deterministic objective approach are both essential in medicine. For this reason (as with holism and mechanistic materialism) an integration of the two approaches is an urgent task for a genuine philosophy of medicine.

In integrating the approaches, the existential principle must be given priority; for the patient must always be treated as a potentially free person. The phenomenological principle is complementary, it considers the sick person's unique individual world intuitively in which he is struggling with the experience of his illness. This framework also allows the doctor to investigate and to treat the patient's body and mind as determined objects. In such a unified, comprehensive approach there is no limit to the employment of different theories and concepts provided that they fulfil the criteria of the scientific method. No single theory can claim a monopoly to absolute truth in science, hence there is no room for sectarianism.

The doctor can treat bodily illness either specifically by means of medicine or surgery, applying the principle of mechanistic-materialism, or unspecifically by means of stimuli which raise the patient's general health, applying the principals of holism. (The latter forms of treatment should always be considered first, as they are in line with nature's own healing efforts and do not entail a risk of dangerous complications or side-effects.)

In the case of mental illness, we saw that the approach of mechanistic materialism is available only for treating the psyche via the brain. The holistic approach was exemplified by the use of unspecific suggestions and of the various methods employed under the name of social psychiatry. The contributions by the traditional schools of analytical psychology had to be re-interpreted in terms of the patient's experience of the challenges of the sexual instinct, the drive for power and such fundamental 'archetypal' experiences as fatherhood, motherhood, God and Devil. In spite of the emphasis on the subjective-ethical principle, it was agreed that the patient and the doctor think in terms of a mental illness, i.e. that they consider the mind as an object which is sick and which, they hope, will recover as the result of the treatment which they both administer in a joint effort. The body plays an important part in mental sickness, as any emotional states of illness often lead to states of bodily sickness, for instance to disturbances of the digestive or respiratory tract or general malaise. The relation between body and mind were considered from the empirical point of view; the body-mind problem, however, turned out to be an insoluble pseudo-problem.

The existential-phenomenological approach involves interpreting to the patient what is going on in his world of experience and especially what his own conscience has to say about the conduct of his life. Clearly, the doctor has to be careful not to impose his own moral views on the patient nor over-tax a person's power of carrying on the struggle for authenticity. He must support the patient battling with physical or mental illness and he must not withhold any physical or mental treatment which is required for relief and is not too harmful through its side-effects. He may even resort to a leucotomy, a brain operation which changes the patient's personality to one which is much more indifferent and therefore does not struggle any more. This is clearly a grave decision to take from the point of view of the doctor's own conscience. But it may have to be faced.

Existential psychotherapy is not a special method which would call for the foundation of yet another school in medicine, rather is it an approach for the doctor who has accepted the principles of Existential

Ethics as binding, whether he is a psychiatrist, a physician, a surgeon or a general practitioner. In that way, the whole of medicine can be humanized.

To render human involves making people aware of their innate moral sense, their conscience, which informs them what they ought to be. The lack of such awareness, I suggest, lies at the root of the anxiety, depression and drug addiction which, as was stated in the Preface, affect one in every five Americans and countless other Western people.

The moral questions which feature in current discussions are mainly concerned with people's rights, with what they ought to *have*: are women entitled to have their unwanted pregnancies terminated, should parents have the freedom to have unborn malformed babies aborted, can patients, suffering from painful terminal illness, demand euthanasia, carried out by doctors, can women, married to sterile husbands, insist to be impregnated by the semen of a donor? While none of these questions can be dismissed as irrelevant from a moral point of view, while the answers to them affect people's lives deeply, they have no direct bearing on people's obligations.

To have a baby can bring fulfilment to a woman, but many women who have children suffer serious nervous breakdowns. They are anxious and depressed and unable to cope with their lives. They form part of the millions covered by the survey of mental health.

Some of these patients are in need of psychotropic drugs such as anti-depressants, they benefit from an application of the science of the brain to the mind. Others benefit from a psychotherapy, but not from its scientific theory.

Hans H. Strupp has demonstrated that there is no evidence that one set of a theoretical framework, underlying a particular form of psycho-therapy, gives better therapeutic results than another set. [119] The same author has found that 'psychotherapeutic change does not depend on the elucidation of historical antecedents' [120] which means that the historical principle of psycho-analysis, quoted earlier [121], is not an essential part of psychotherapy. Patients do not have to be regressed to early childhood, the 'cause' of their illness has not be traced to its 'origin'. As Strupp has pointed out, the personal relationship with the therapist is the vital element in the treatment which agrees with the view discussed already.

The role of the therapist is defined by K. Mitchell and his co-workers and they confirm further the validity of the libertarian-exististential approach: The essential requirements for a successful treatment therapist are 1) empathy or intuition, 2) non-possessive warmth and

3) genuineness [122]. These findings are in agreement with the conditions which, we saw, must be fulfilled so that a therapist can meet his patient in the psychotherapeutic encounter.

NOTES

[1] 'Human Relations in Obstetric Practice', *Lancet*, 23 April 1960, pp. 913-15.

[2] ibid, p. 915.

[3] ibid, p. 915.

[4] Leading Article, *Brit. Med. J.*, 16 May, 1964, p. 1267.

[5] See 'Mortality in Relation to Smoking: Ten Years' Observations of British Doctors', *Brit. Med. J.*, 30 May 1964, pp. 1399-410.

[6] *Behaviour Therapy and the Neuroses*, edited by H. J. Eysenck, Pergamon Press, Oxford, London, New York, Paris, 1960, p. 19.

[7] *Sigmund Freud, Life and Work*, vol. 3, 1955, London, The Hogarth Press, p. 329.

[8] ibid.

[9] ibid, pp. 329-30.

[10] *Group Psychology and the Analysis of the Ego*, 1921, Engl. transl. London, The Hogarth Press, 1955, vol. 18, p. 90.

[11] ibid, p. 111,

[12] ibid.

[13] E. Fromm, *Man for Himself*, London, 1950, Routledge & Kegan Paul, pp. 144-5.

[14] ibid, p. 156.

[15] ibid, p. 157.

[16] ibid, p. 158.

[17] *The Archetypes and the Collective Unconscious*, ibid, vol. 9, p. 79.

[18] *Instinct and the Unconscious, Contributions to Analytical Psychology* by C. G. Jung, Engl. trans. London, 1928, Kegan Paul, Trench, Trubner & Co. Ltd., p. 276.

[19] *The Integration of the Personality*, by C. G. Jung, Engl. transl. London, Kegan Paul, Trench, Trubner & Co., 1940, p. 80.

[20] ibid.

[21] *Die Beziehungen zwischen dem Ich und dem Unbewussten*, Rascher & Co. Zürich, Leipzig und Stuttgart, 1933, p. 179.

[22] C. G. Jung, *Memories, Dreams, Reflections*, recorded and edited by Aniela Jaffé, English transl., Collins, and Routledge & Kegan Paul, London, 1963, p. 179.

[23] C. G. Jung, *Die Beziehungen zwischen dem Ich und dem Umbewussten*, Rascher & Co., Zürich, Leipzig und Stuttgart, 1933, p. 182.

[24] ibid.

[25] See *Memories, Dreams, Reflections,* by C. G. Jung, recorded and edited by Aniela Jaffé, Engl. transl., Collins and Routledge & Kegan Paul, London, 1963.

[26] *The Archetypes and the Collective Unconscious,* Kegan Paul, Coll. Works, vol. 9, p. 275.

[27] Hans Trüb, *Heilung aus der Begegnung,* Ernst Klett Verlag, Stuttgart, 1951, p. 80.

[28] ibid, p. 40.

[29] ibid, p. 32.

[30] Philip Rieff, 'C. G. Jung's Confessions, Psychology as a Language of Faith', *Encounter,* May 1964, pp. 49-50.

[31] It is essential to distinguish between Husserl's phenomenological method and his philosophy of 'pure phenomenology' which is unacceptable, for Husserl's 'pure phenomenology' claims to provide absolute knowledge, in the form of an 'eidetic science', established without having recourse to empirical observation.

[32] *Ideas, General Introduction to Pure Phenomenology,* English transl. London, 1931, George Allen & Unwin Ltd., New York, The Macmillan Company, p. 113.

[33] P. Foulquié, *Existentialism,* Engl. transl. Dennis Dobson Ltd., 1948, p. 49.

[34] The term 'existential psychiatrist' here and elsewhere is not meant to include all those psychiatrists who call themselves existential, but is used to designate the particular approach adopted in this book.

[35] The difference between the doctor and the philosopher has already been mentioned; it is illustrated in this instance by the existential philosopher and the existential psychiatrist, concerned on the one hand with theoretical formulation only and on the other with the effects which the holding of certain values has on the person's health.

[36] Francis A. Macnab, *Estrangement and Relationship,* 1964, Tavistock Publications, London, p. 221.

[37] Helen Merrel Lynd, *On Shame and the Search for Identity,* quoted in paper by Maurice Friedman, 'Existential Psychotherapy and the Image of Man', *J. of Humanistic Psychology,* Fall 1964, p. 114.

[38] See p. 127.

[39] *The Divided Self,* R. D. Laing, Tavistock Publications, London, 1960.

[40] ibid.

[41] ibid, p. 45.

[42] ibid, p. 47.

[43] ibid, p. 48.

[44] Husserl spoke of 'grades of giveness or clearness' and of the possibility of 'enhancing the clearness of what is already intuitable'. See his *Ideas, General Introduction to Pure Phenomenology*, London, 1931, George Allen & Unwin Ltd., New York, The Macmillan Company, pp. 195-6. It could, therefore, be said that bringing material from the unconscious into the conscious mind amounts to bringing data of consciousness from the dark into the light, from an unclear into a clear position.

[45] *The Self and Others*, Tavistock Publications, 1961, London, p. 21.

[46] R. D. Laing has described this situation in *The Self and Others*, pp. 155-70.

[47] *The Emotions*, English transl. Philosophical Library, New York, 1949, pp. 58, 90.

[48] Oxford University Press, 7th ed., 1950.

[49] ibid, p. 210.

[50] ibid.

[51] ibid, p. 231.

[52] *The Case of Ellen West*, Engl. transl. *Existence*, Basic Books, 1958, pp. 237-364.

[53] ibid, p. 256.

[54] *Findings in a Case of Schizophrenic Depression*, English transl. ibid, pp. 127-38.

[55] ibid, p. 133.

[56] Psychiatrists, interested in a phenomenological analysis of their patients, have examined these distortions systematically. See, for instance, H. F. Ellenberger, *A Clinical Introduction to Psychiatric Phenomenology and Existential Analysis*, ibid, pp. 92-124. Such studies are not concerned with conceptual scientific frameworks, only with subjective experiences, all tinted with emotions.

[57] 7th ed. Oxford University Press, 1950, p. 299.

[58] *The Divided Self*, Tavistock Publications, 1960, London, p. 170.

[59] *The Self and Others*, Tavistock Publications, London, 1961, pp. 90-7.

[60] The insight into the existential root of schizophrenic illness does not rule out that there might be other explanations such as abnormalities in the person's brain which were referred to in the introduction to this section and which requires physical treatment.

[61] *The Emotions*, English transl., Philosophical Library, New York, 1948, pp. 66, 67.

[62] See V. E. v. Gebsattel, *Prolegomena einer medizinschen Anthropologie*, Springer-Verlag, Berlin Göttingen-Heidelberg, 1954, pp. 183-200.

[63] K. Jaspers has stressed this aspect of Freud's work in his *General Psychopathology*, Eng. transl. from the German 7th ed., Manchester University Press, 1963.

[64] Hans Trüb, *Heilung aus der Begegnung*, Ernst Klett Verlag, 1951, p. 59.

[65] C. G. Jung, *Instinct and the Unconscious, Contributions to Analytical Psychology*, Eng. transl., London, 1940, Kegan Paul, Trench, Trubner & Co., p. 80.

[66] *The Individual Psychology of Alfred Adler*, edited and annotated by Heinz L. Ansbacher and Rowan R. Ansbacher, New York, Basic Books, Inc., 1956, pp. 397-8.

[67] The above criticism does not invalidate Adler's insight into the striving for superiority which a child might well express by an attempt to tyrannize its family. In the case quoted, the anxiety which the little girl is reported to have felt must be judged as genuine and not put on, and therefore Adler's interpretation and treatment must be considered to have been contrary to the existential standpoint.

[68] *Nausea*, A New Directions Paperbook, U.S.A., 1959, p. 210.

[69] ibid, p. 173.

[70] ibid, p. 209.

[71] Eng. transl. Methuen & Co. Ltd., 1957.

[72] *Being and Nothingness*, p. 364.

[73] ibid, p. 621.

[74] ibid. p. 464.

[75] *Being and Time*, Eng. transl. 1962, SCM Press Ltd., London, p. 223.

[76] *What Makes Us Behave at all Socially?*, Review of Existential Psychology and Psychiatry, 1964, vol. 4, no. 1, p. 63.

[77] ibid, p. 59.

[78] M. Boss, *Psychoanalyse und Daseinsanalytik*, Hans Huber, Bern und Stuttgart, 1957, p. 99.

[79] The terms 'fundamental' and 'regional' ontology are quotations from Husserl's system of pure phenomenology which was earlier rejected as a basis for an existential medical ethics. It is ironic that Boss has found in Heidegger the true exponent of Husserlian philosophy, whereas Husserl himself repudiated Heidegger's interpretation of his phenomenology.

[80] *The Sickness Unto Death*, Doubleday Anchor Books, New York, 1954, p. 201.

[81] *Fear and Trembling*, Doubleday Anchor Books, New York, 1954, p. 48.

[82] See Kierkegaard's *Fear and Trembling*, published with *The Sickness unto Death* in Doubleday Anchor Books, New York, 1954.

[83] Eng. transl. published by Hamish Hamilton, London, 1955.

[84] ibid, p. 99.

[85] Penguin Books, 1960.

[86] ibid, p. 178.

[87] ibid, p. 108.

[88] *Reason and Existence*, The Noonday Press, 1957, p. 141.

[89] *Man in the Modern Age*, Eng. transl., Routledge & Kegan Paul, Ltd., 1951, p. 78.

[90] *The Perennial Scope of Philosophy*, Philosophical Library, New York, 1949, pp. 181, 182.

[91] ibid, p. 46.

[92] *I and Thou*, 2nd edition, Eng. transl., T. & T. Clark, Edinburgh, 1959, p. 76.

[93] *The Perennial Scope of Philosophy*, p. 167.

[94] *Between Man and Man*, Kegan Paul, London, 1947, p. 178.

[95] *I and Thou*, 2nd edition, Eng. transl., T. & T. Clark, Edinburgh, 1959, p. 70.

[96] See p. 139.

[97] John A. T. Robinson, *The New Reformation?*, S.C.M. Press Ltd., London, 1965, p. 32.

[98] M. Buber, *I and Thou*, 2nd edition, Eng. transl., T. & T. Clark, Edinburgh, 1959, p. 106.

[99] *Martin Buber, Guilt and Guilt Feelings*, The William Alanson White Memorial Lectures, *Psychiatry*, vol. 20, no. 2, 1957, p. 117.

[100] In Buber's essay, quoted earlier, existential guilt is distinguished from the guilt which he describes as 'neurotic' and 'groundless'. — The latter is exemplified by 'repressed childhood wishes and youthful lust gone astray', whereas the former is illustrated by 'the inner consequences of a man's betrayal of his friend or his cause'. Buber admits that both forms are 'intermingled'. In establishing the presence of guilt, it is obviously important to establish the degree of consciousness or unconsciousness, as a person can be considered (by himself or by others) as 'guilty' only if he could have acted differently, i.e. if he was conscious of the moral significance of his action. (Allowance must be made for half-awareness which may manifest itself in feelings of uneasiness.) Apart from existential guilt, incurred by injuring others, there is the guilt of not having fulfilled one's obligations to oneself, of not having succeeded in establishing an authentic self. It is the recognition of this guilt, evident in the patient's own 'bad conscience', which provides the basis for existential psychology. For further clarification of the question of authentic and neurotic guilt, see H. Fingerette, 'Real Guilt and Neurotic Guilt', *J. of Existential Psychiatry*, vol. 3, no. 10, 1962, pp. 145-58.

[101] E. Herzog, *Psyche und Tod*, Rascher Verlag, Zürich und Stuttgart, 1960, pp. 160-1.

[102] Doubleday Anchor Books, New York, 1954.

[103] ibid, p. 153.

[104] Martin Buber, *Postcript, I and Thou*, 2nd edition, T. & T. Clark, Edinburgh, 1959, p. 133.

[105] See C. A. Seguin, *Love and Psychotherapy, The Psychotherapeutic Eros, Acta psychother.*, 10, 1962, pp. 187, 190.

[106] W. Dilthey, *Das Verstehen anderer Personen, und ihrer Lebensäusserungen, Gesammelte Werke*, Bd. 7, Teubner, Leipzig u. Berlin, 1927, p. 214.

[107] Vol. 3, no. 473, April 1965.

[108] Karl Jaspers, *General Psychopathology*, Eng. transl. from the German, 7th edition, 1962, Manchester University Press, pp. 302-3.

[109] A patient may become aware, for instance, of his sexual desire or his intellectural or artistic abilities as a result of existential psychotherapy.

[110] V. E. v. Gebsattel, *Prolegomena einer medizinishen Anthropologie*, Springer Verlag, Berlin, Göttingen, Heidelberg, 1954, p. 277.

[111] See M. Scheler, *Das Ressentiment im Aufbau der Moralen*, Gesammelte Werke, Band 3, 4. Aufl. Francke Verlag, Bern, 1934.

[112] For a survey of the applications of existential psychotherapy see Ledermann, E. K., *Mental Health and Human Conscience: The True and False Self*, Gower, 1985.

[113] W. A. Luijpen, *Existential Phenomenology*, 1963, Duquesne University Press, Pittsburgh, Pa., pp. 186, 187.

[114] *The Image and Appearance of the Human Body*, Psyche Monographs, No. 4, 1935, Kegan Paul, Trench, Trubner & Co., p. 143.

[115] ibid.

[116] ibid, p. 287.

[117] ibid, p. 283.

[118] *The Autogene Training, a Psychophysiological Approach in Psychotherapy*, Grune & Stratton, New York 1959.

[119] H. H. Strupp, 'A Reformulation of the Dynamics of the Therapist's Contribution' chapter 1, *Effective Psychotherapy: A Handbook of Research*, Pergamon Press 1977, p. 10.

[120] ibid, p. 17.

[121] See pp. 81-83.

[122] K. M. Mitchell and others, 'A Reappraisal of the Therapeutic Effectiveness of Accurate Empathy, Nonpossessive Warmth and Genuineness', chapter 18, *Effective Psychotherapy*, p. 483.

Author Index

Adler, A., 76, 83, 84, 85, 86, 143, 144, 145
Adler, G., 88, 105n, 106n
Ansbacher, H. L. and R. R., 83, 105n
Aristotle, 34, 52
Avery-Jones, F., xxii
Ayer, A. J., 51, 60n

Bardon, D., 99, 100, 101
Baudouin, C., 29, 94
Berkeley, Bishop, 55
Bierer, J., 38n
Binswanger, L., 139
Blanchard, B., xix, xxiv
Boole, G., 112
Boss, M., 148, 149, 168
Bowlby, J., 100
Bridgman, P. W., 53, 54, 55, 61n
Broad, A. C., 71
Buber, M., 70, 152, 155, 169, 170n
Burnet, Sir MacFarlane, 19, 20, 36, 37n

Campbell, G. D., xxii, xxiii, 37n, 140
Camus, A., 149, 150
Cannon, W. B., 19, 36
Cassirer, E., 77, 78
Cleave, T. L., xxi, xxii, xxiii, 26, 37n
Collingwood, R. G., xix, xxiv, 3, 10, 16
Copernicus, 44
Coué, E., 28, 29
Crick, F. H. C., 21, 37n
Crookshank, F. G., 111

Dilthey, W., 76, 77, 155, 170n
Doll, R., xxii, 27
Driesch, H., 34, 37n
Durnin, J. V. G. A., 37n

Ellenberger, H. F., 140, 167n
Erikson, E. H., 70

Fairbairn, W. R. D., 79
Fenichel, O., 22, 37n, 80, 104, 105n, 106n
Fessard, A. E., 51, 60n
Fingerette, H., 168n

Fordham, F., 93, 106n
Fordham, M., 87, 88, 89, 92, 93, 106n
Foulkes, S. H., 32
Foulquié, P., 129, 166n
Frankl, V. E., 129
Frege, G., 112
Freud, S., 22, 23, 76, 77, 78, 82, 83, 94, 104n, 110, 123, 124, 125, 135, 143, 165n
Friedman, M., 166n
Fromm, E., 125, 165n

Galen, 52
Gebsattel, V. E. von, 142, 166n, 170n
Giel, R., Knox, R. S. and Carstairs, G. M., 101, 108n
Goethe, J. W. von, 127
Gordon, R. E. and K. E., 67
Grinker, R. G. Sr., 63, 64, 65
Grünfeld, B., 67
Guntrip, H., 23-4, 104n, 111, 114n

Haldane, J. S., 56
Harvey, W., 112
Hawkins, N. G., 73-4, 75, 104n
Heidegger, M., 146, 148, 151, 152, 159
Henderson, D. and Gillespie, R. D., 138, 139, 140, 141
Herzog, E., 153, 155, 170n
Hes, J. Ph., 67
Hill, A., 30, 38n
Hoff, E. C. and Riese, W., 52, 61n
Hopkins, F. G., 10
Hunt, J. McVicker, 96-7, 107n
Huntling, I., 38
Husserl, E., 128, 129, 130, 166n, 167n, 168n

Jacobi, J., 87, 105n, 106n
Jackson, M., 89, 90, 106n
Jaspers, K., 57, 58, 62, 78, 79, 90, 91, 95, 103n, 106n, 150, 151, 152, 155, 168n, 170n
Jeans, Sir James, 45, 55, 60n
Johnson, Dr., 55
Jones, E., 110, 123
Jones, M., 75
Jung, C. G., 76, 77, 87, 88, 89, 92, 94, 104n, 105n, 106n, 126, 127, 128, 143, 165n, 166n, 168n

Kant, I., 44, 45, 46, 50, 54, 57, 58,
  60n, 61n, 62, 66, 71, 72, 75, 76,
  79, 85, 86, 92, 102n, 104n
Kapp, R. O., 17, 18, 37n
Kierkegaard, S., 149, 155, 168n
Klein, M., 79

Laing, R. D., 134, 141, 154, 166n,
  167n, 168n
Landé, A., 55
Ledermann, E. K., 38n, 170n
Leff, J., 68, 103n
Lorenz, K., 70, 71, 103n
Lujpen, W. A., 161, 170n
Lynd, H. M., 130, 166n

Macnab, F. A., 130, 166n
Mannheim, K., 78, 79, 104n
Martin, M. E., 100
Medawar, Sir Peter, 10, 20, 21, 25, 37n
Mendel, G., 20
Meredith, J. C., 58, 61n
Meyer, A., 110
Minkowski, E., 140
Mitchell, K. M., 164, 165, 170n
Morris, N., 120, 121
McDougall, W., 93, 111
McCarrison, Sir Robert, xxiii

Nagel, E., 4, 5, 7, 18, 67, 68, 69, 73,
  107n
Neuer, A., 86

Ogden, C. K. and Richards, I. A., 111,
  114n

Papanoutsos, E. P., 82
Pavlov, I., 11, 12, 51
Popper, Sir Karl, 46, 60n, 112
Pucetti, R., 51

Rennie, T. A. C., 31, 38n
Rieff, P., 128, 166n
Riese, W., 52, 61n
Robinson, J. A. T., 153, 169n
Rollier, A., 30
Rosenbluth, A., Wiener, N. and
  Bigelow, J., 7
Russell, Bertrand, 109

Salvesen, C., 67
Sartre, J.-P., 136, 137, 138, 141, 146,
  147, 151, 157
Scheler, M., 170n
Schilder, P., 161, 170n
Schultz, J. H., 161, 162, 170n
Seguin, C. A., 155, 170n
Slavson, S. R., 32
Smuts, J., xxi, 16, 17, 37n, 43, 47, 84
Spitz, R., 100
Straus, E., 12
Strupp, H. H., 164, 170n
Sullivan, H. S., 71, 103n
Swanson, J. W., 9

Taylor, C., 95, 96, 97
Thompson, K. M., 127, 128, 166n,
  168n
Trüb, H., 126, 127, 165n, 167n

Vaihinger, H., 85, 86, 145

Watson, J. B., 11, 15
Way, L., 85, 86
White, W., 97, 98, 107n
Windelband, W., 86
Wolpe, J., 11, 12, 13n
Woodger, J. H., 35, 109, 113, 115n

Young, J. Z., 6, 8, 9, 21, 58, 59-60

Subject Index

abreaction, 159
action
    behavioural definition of, 64, 65
    in contrast to movement, 95, 96, 97
activity, psychic, 90, 95
Adlerian psychology, 76, 83-6, 92,
    143-5
Adler's Place in Psychology, 85
adopted child, 66
aggression, 27, 28, 79
aggressiveness, 69, 78, 79, 80
aggressive object relations, theory of, 80
alcohol, effects of, 52, 70, 93
Alcoholics Anonymous, 70
analgesics, 34, 161
analogy, use of, 7, 8, 10, 20, 57, 58, 64
analyst's expectations, 79
analytical-specific approach, xxi
anger, xiv, 5, 29, 51, 73, 86, 139, 161
anima, 88, 94, 126, 127
animal, identification of man and, 52
animus, 88, 94
antibodies, 10, 19, 35, 68
anti-social behaviour, 69, 154
aptitude tests, 98
archetypal contents of unconscious,
    127
archetypal energy, 88
archetypal experiences, 145, 164
archetypal power, 89, 90
archetypal self, 128
archetypal theory, 87-8, 93, 126
as-if, philosophy of, 145
association of ideas, 95
atom(s), 9, 16, 17, 18, 19, 36, 45
atomic holism, 19
atomic model, 17
authenticity, 130, 133, 135, 148, 151,
    160, 164, *see also* self, healthy,
    true
authority, 125
auto-immune diseases, 19, 20

Being and Nothingness, 147, 157
'Behavior, Purpose and Teleology', 7
behaviour, 5, 63, 69, 95
behaviour therapy, 13, 122-3
behavioural science a comprehensive,
    63-5

behaviourism, 22, 63, 110
behaviourist(ic) theory, 13, 16
behaviourists, 11, 50
biological phenomena, 57, 59, 68, 109,
    110
biological reality, 56
Biological Retrospect, A, 10, 25
biological substrate, 87
biological-instinctual interpretation of
    maternity, 101
biological-psychiatric determinism, 101
biologism, 109, 110
biolo-psychologism, 110, 111
biology, significance of holism and
    mechanistic materialism in,
    56-60
bodily disease, *see* bodily illness
bodily functions, 72
bodily health, 28, 74
bodily illness, xxi, 25-8, 34, 141, 163,
    164
bodily maintenance, 73
bodily movement, 96
bodily phenomena, 64, 90
body
    and mind, relation of, 49-53, 54,
        62, 96, 164
    as opposed to mind, xix, xxi, 5, 18,
        19, 22, 30, 32, 36, 44, 47, 48,
        56, 64, 65, 68, 72, 75, 76, 83,
        90, 93, 95, 98, 99, 101, 112,
        128, 159, 163
    the experience of the, 161-3
boredom, 97, 146
brain, the, 5, 6, 7, 8, 9, 50, 51, 52, 53,
    58, 88, 92, 93, 98, 137, 162,
    164
    teleology in Young's conception of,
        59-60, 143
breast-feeding, 80
Buddhist teachings, 153

Cantor Lectures (1936), xxiii
carbohydrates, refined, xxi, xxii, xxiii,
    27
Cartesian dualism, 161
categories of understanding, 44, 54
catharsis, 32

173

causality, 44, 45, 49, 81, 82, 83, 85, 86, 140
causal principle, the, 132
Central and Scottish Health Services Council, 121
cerebral phenomena, 60
challenge
    of instinctual urges, 145
    life as a, 119, 126, 127, 133, 141
    of physical illness, 161
    of the sexual urge, 142, 164
    social, 65-7, 70, 71, 72, 73, 75, 76, 137
children, disturbed, 31
children, group treatment of, 32
Christ, 91
Christian teachings, 153
chromosomes, 70
code, 6, 21, 25, 29
cognition, 72, 95
collective social mind, the, 66, 73
collective unconsious, the, 87, 88, 90, 91, 143
collusion, 136
communication, 64, 151, 152, 153, 158
    community psychiatry, 67, 70
comparative mythology, 92
competence, 97
compulsive-obsessional, the, 137-8, 150
computers, 6, 8, 9, 18, 20, 59
concept(s)
    as a tool, 114
    constitutive, 56
    and physical reality, 53-5
conflict, xx, 22, 24, 28, 67, 75, 131, 138, 149, 157
congruity, 149
conscience, 75, 81, 98, 119, 125, 129, 130, 131, 135, 138, 141, 154, 164
consciousness, 51, 89, 129, 130, 135, 139, 143, 147, 159
constitutive judgement, 57, 58
contingency, 147
Copernican Revolution, the, 43-5, 50, 56, 58, 60, 62, 114
coronary disease, xxi, xxii, xxiv, 27, 121
counterhomeostatic behaviour, 23
courage, 86, 97, 126, 161, 163
Critique of Pure Reason, The, 62
Critique of Teleological Judgement, The, 57, 58
crowd mentality, 148
culture, significance of, 70
Current Perspectives in Social Psychology, 96

Darwinism, 84

data of consciousness, 130, 135, 143
death, fear of, 51
'death' of God, 129, 145
death instinct, 23, 78, 79, 80
delinquents, 84
delusions, 76, 90, 91, 94, 126
deoxyribonucleic acid (DNA), 4, 20
depersonalization, 94, 162
depression, 32, 49, 52, 67, 76, 78, 80, 119, 132, 133, 137
depressive, the, 138-9
Designer, the, 43, 46, 47
despair, 129, 146, 149, 150, 157
destructive urge, 79, 135, 147
determinant judgement, 57
determinism, xix, xx, xxiv, 4, 22, 68, 81, 83, 85, 98, 99, 101, 102, see also mechanistic determinism
deterministic approach, 132
deterministic explanation, 21
deterministic language, 101
deterministic material-holistic conception, 23
deterministic-mechanistic treatment, xxi
deterministic principle, 44, 99
deterministic psychologies, 122-8
deterministic-objective approach, 163
deterministic pattern, 16
deterministic-scientific approach to social life, 68-9, 70
developmental approach to social evolution, 71
Diabetes, Coronary Thrombosis and the Saccharine Disease, xxii, xxiv
dialogical relationship, 152, 153
dietetic treatment, xxi, 26, 27, 32
Dionysius, 91
disease, see bodily, coronary, iatrogenic, infectious, mental, paradontal
disturbed children, 31
Divided Self, The, 134
doctor-patient relationship, the, 119-20ff.
dreams, 88, 90, 92, 158
drugs, xx, 26, 32, 33, 93, 99, 101, 109, 132, 139, 159
dualism
    Cartesian, 161
    Jungian, 89
duodenal ulcer, xx, xxi, xxiii, xxiv, 26, 49

effectance motivation, 98
efficient causality, 83
ego, 22, 23, 24, 28, 78, 81, 89, 94
electro-convulsions, 99, 139
electron, 3, 45, 55
embryology, 25

emotion(s), 5, 10, 51, 52, 136, 137, 138, 141
emotional cravings, xxii
emotional disabilities, 49
emotional disturbances, 49, 66
emotional factors, xx
emotional illness, 30, 67, 76, 100
emotional ties, 23
empirical reality, 54
endocrine glands, 27, 87, 92
energy
    archetypal, 88
    concept of, 4, 35, 46, 54
    emotional, 159
    libidinal, 23, 110, 126
energy principal, the, 3
engineering, language of, 6, 8, 59
engulfment, 134, 154
entelechy, 34, 35
entropy, 46
environment, 12, 36, 65, 67, 78, 96, 97, 132, 133
environmental treatments, holistic, 30-4, 47, 65
epidemiological psychiatric knowledge, 67-8
epistemological conclusions re individual medical psychology, 92-4
epistemological evaluation of Jungian psychology, 90-2
ethical approach, 70, 72, 75
ethical principle, 143, 145
ethical problems, 75
ethics, 44, 52, 109, 110, 111, 114, 119-65, 165, and passim
evolution, 16, 70-1
evolutionary teleology, 84
existence, 130
existential and phenomenological principles, integration of, 130-42
existential ethical principle, the, 130
existential ethics
    medicine and, 128-63
    medicine based on, 163-5
existential guilt, 153, 154
existential ontologies, 130, 145
existential phenomenological approach, 163, 164
existential re-interpretation of traditional medical psychologies, 142
existential (psycho) therapy, 130, 149-60
existentialism, 129
exhibitionism, 142

fallacy of the deterministic-scientific approach to social life, 68-9
family, 31, 66, 73, 136
faith, 145-6, 149, 150, 151ff.
fear, 5, 29, 51, 70, 97
fetishism, 46

free association, 158
free will, 44, 121
freedom, 65, 66, 69-70, 94-9, 100, 102, 121-36 passim, 143-50 passim, 157, 160
    of social actions, 70-1
    psychic determinism and, 94-9
Freudian psychology, xx, xxi, 22, 64, 76-83, 88, 92, 123-6, 142-3
frigidity, 124

gastric ulcer, xx, xxi, 74
genetic factor, xx, 87, 98, 121
genetics, 21, 25, 64, 70, 93, 137
Gestalt psychology, 95, 162
goals, 16, 85
God
    as archetype, 88, 91
    'death' of, 129, 145
    existence of, 46-7
    faith in, 149
    in Jungian psychology, 127
    search for, 153
    union with, 159
Greek papyrus and solar penis, 91
guilt, 80, 98, 125, 131, 138, 139, 144, 153, 154
gynaecologists, 161

hallucinations, 88, 94
hatred, 73, 79, 80, 139, 153
health, xxi, xxii, 18, 22, 24, 28, 32, 52, 65, 72, 73, 74, 93, 121, 128, 131, 132
heart, the, 8, 10, 18, 32, 57, 95
hedonism, 126
hedonistic ethical view, 131
Heidegger's ontology, 148-9
hermeneutic principle, 76-8, 81
hermeneutic-naturalistic historical determinism, 83
'Hermeneutik, Die Entstehung der', 77
heuristic function of models, 7
heuristic principle, 57
historical causality, 82
historical knowledge, 82
historical principle, the, 76, 81-3
historical time, 82
historical-libidinal determinism, 81
holism
    in physics and biology, 17-21
    its relationship with mechanistic materialism, 56-60
    Jungian, 89-90
    the philosophy of, 16-37
holistic agent, 34
holistic approach, the, xxi, xxii, xxiii, xxiv, 5, 50
holistic conception, the, 84
holistic environmental treatments, 30-4, 65

holistic feature in life, 114
holistic forces in body, 48
holistic power, 35
holistic principle, the, 4, 24-5
    and the material substrate, 34-6
    in medical practice, 25-34
holistic processes, 6, 90
holistic suggestion, 28-9
homeostasis, 19, 23, 24, 83
homeostatic mechanisms, 35, 36, 64
homeostats, 6, 8, 17, 20, 59
homosexuality, 142
human nature, 77, 81, 90
human relations, evaluation of in
    medical psychology, 99-102
human relationships, 70, 127, 153, 154
Husserlian phenomenology, 128-9, 135,
    143
hypochondria, 67, 162
hypostatization, 46, 48, 62, 113
hysteria, 132
hysterical psychoses, 67, 101
hysteric, the, 141-2, 148, 151

I and Thou, 153
iatrogenic diseases, 33
id, 78
idealism, 3
idea, the, as an expression of meta-
    physical thought, 63, 75
ideas, association of, 95
identification, 23, 124
identity, personal, 62, 75
idiographic science, 86
illegitimate child, 66
illness, xxi, xxii, 3, 19, 22, 25-34, 35,
    47, 48, 49, 67, 76, 77, 78, 93,
    98, 100, 122, 123, 129, 131,
    132, 133, 141, 163, 164
immunization, 26
implosion, 134, 154
impotence, 124
indeterminism, 45
individual, the, xix, xxiv, 16, 22, 23,
    47, 65, 66, 68, 70, 75, 76, 81,
    82, 85, 86, 87, 89, 98, 101,
    125, 127, 128
individual mind, the, 73
individual phenomena, 68
Individual Psychology of Alfred Adler,
    The, see also Alderian Psycho-
    logy
individuality, 95, 120
individuation, 89, 127
infectious diseases, 26, 35
inferiority, 49, 85, 144, 145
information, significance of, 6, 8, 21,
    25, 36, 64
insecurity, 66, 134, 146, 151
instinct(s), 10, 23, 79, 87, 92, 111
instinctual determinism, 126

instinctual development, 79
instinctual disturbance, 143, 144, 148,
    163
instinctual energy, 22, 78, 142
instinctual gratification, 77
instinctual libido, xxi, 124
instinctual patterns, 70, 87
instinctual urges, 75, 146
intelligence tests, 98
inter-human order, 154
inter-human relations, 73, 153
Interpersonal Theory of Psychiatry,
    The, 71
interpersonal relations, 71, 72
introversion, 157
invasion-healing processes, 89-90
irrational determinism, 126
isolation, 68

Jewish teachings, 153
Jungian dualism, 89
Jungian ontology, 87-8
Jungian psychology, 86-92, 126-7, 143

Kantian epistemology, passim
    and psychological medicine, 62,102
    and science, 43-60
    and the unification of scientific
        thought, 109-14
knowledge, 44, 45, 50, 53, 55, 56, 57,
    63, 76, 82, 83, 91, 113, 130,
    155

learning, 11-12, 16
leucotomy, 163
libertarian approach, 132
libertarian language, 101
libertarian principle, the, 99, 102
libidinal energy, 23, 110, 126
libidinal object relationship, 80
libidinal satisfaction, 120
libidinal theory, 10
libido, xxi, 79, 81, 88, 93, 124
life, creation of, 110
life instinct, 23
'Logic Without Assumptions', 112
love, 123, 141, 154, 155
lungs, 18, 101

machine(s), 5, 6, 7, 8, 16, 17, 20, 25,
    36, 58, 59, 60, 78
Man and Society, 78
mandalas, 89, 91, 127
manic, the, 139, 150, 153
marriages, unhappy, 136
masochistic activities, 23
masochistic phenomena, 78
mass, concept of, 54
masturbation, 142
materialism, 16, 63, 109
materialistic machinist, 35

materialistic thesis, 52
matrix, concept of the, 74
mechanisms, xix, xxi, xxii, 36, 72, 74, 95, 96, 98
mechanistic argument, xxiv
mechanistic determinism, 69
mechanistic materialism, xx, xxi, xxiv, 3-15, 17, 20, 36, 43, 44, 46, 49, 50, 56-60, 62, 69, 114, 120, 212, 163, 164
mechanistic-materialistic approach, the, 32
mechanists, 24, 25, 26
medical judgement, 24, 25, 26
Medical Sociology, Theory, Scope and Method, 74
medicine
    and ethics, 119-65
    and existential ethics, 128-63
    and naturalistic ethics, 120-28
    based on existential ethics, 163-5
    psychological theory in, 62-3
memory, 8, 60
mental abnormalities, 93
mental health, 21, 73, 74
Mental Health Films, 159
mental illness, 28-34, 98, 99, 132, 144
mental object, 95
mental patient, society's attitude to, 69-70
mental phenomena, theory of, 62, 65, 96, 97, 98
metaphysical doctrine, 110, 112
metaphysical entity, 109
metaphysical theory, 62
methodology, 109
mind, relation of body to, 49-53, 54, 62, 63, 96, 164
modality, 44
model, the, in physico-chemical materialism, 7-10, 14n
'molecular' or 'molar' responses, 11
molecules, 16, 17, 19, 20, 21, 36
momentum, concept of, 54
monistic biological mechanistic materialism, 10-13
monistic physico-chemical materialism, 3-7
monological relationship, 152
moral acts and intentions, 130
moral character of self, 143
moral conflict, 131
moral dimension, man's, 126
moral judgement, 73, 131, 135
moral philosophy, 120, 128
moral point of view, 82, 98, 119, 131
moral principle, the, 71, 97, 102, 125
moral struggle, 163
moral valuation, 80
morphogenesis, 25

mother-baby relationship, 79-80, 99-101, 111
mother-child relationship, 71-2
'Motivation Reconsidered: the Concept of Competence', 97
motives, 97, 98
movement, definition of, 95, 96
mutuality, 152
Myth of Sisyphus, The, 149
myths, 90, 126

naive realism and the naive realistic approach, 43, 47, 49, 50, 52, 53, 54, 56, 57, 58, 59, 62, 65, 76, 78, 81, 82, 86, 90, 114
'naked ape, the', 70
naturalistic determinism, 143
naturalistic-biological principle, the, 76, 78-81, 82
naturalistic ethics, medicine and, 120-28
naturalistic-scientific approach, 70, 83
natural phenomena, 56, 57
natural selection, 71
natural therapy, 27, 30, 33, 34, 48
Nausea, 146, 147
neo-Freudians, 23, 79, 80, 111
nervous breakdown, 132, 133, 149
nervous system, 11, 24, 54, 87, 88, 92, 96, 98
neural explanation of mental phenomena, 96
neurones, 88
neurosis, 90, 129
    symptoms, 22, 142
neurotic(s), 31, 32, 77, 79, 84, 85, 144, 151, 152, 154, 161
neurotic illness, 77, 121, 125
nexus effectivus, 58
nexus finalis, 58
nexus, social, 136
nominalism, 111, 112, 113
nomothetic science, 86
non-deterministic non-scientific approach, 96
non-naturalistic ethics, 84, 127
non-ontological positive existential philosophies, 149-54
'noogenic' neurosis, 129
nosological diagnosis, 100

obesity, 49
object(s)
    exciting or rejecting, theory of, 111
    found in nature, 56
    metaphysical, 62
    of knowledge, 45, 50, 76
    of natural science, psyche as, 78, 83, 90, 92
    patient as, 120-28
    of science, 44, 62, 76, 96, 98

transcendental, 44
object conversion, 46, 62
object relations, 23-4
objective knowledge, 90
objective values, 129
objective-naturalistic science, 86
objective teleology, 86
objective-theoretical approach, 80
obsession, 133, 137-8
occupational therapy, 30, 31
octopus, 6, 59
Oedipus, 124
On Aggression, 70
ontological metaphysics, 44
ontological structure of universe, 43
ontology
    Jungian, 77-8
    of Sartre and Heidegger, 146-9
oral frustration, xx
organic approach in psychiatry, 93
organic reality, 110
Osiris, 91
other, the, 147, 151

pain, xx, 12, 51
paradontal disease, xxi, 27
paranoia, 154
paranoid psychoses, 67
paranoid schizophrenia, 140
paranoids, 162
pathological-psychiatric determinism,
    101
patient, the
    as object, 120-28
    as subject, 128-63
    his struggle for faith, 145-6
    moral strength of, 137
    relationship with doctor, 119-20
    sense of values of, 123, 124, 128
Peptic Ulcer, The, xxiii, xxiv
perception, 43, 95
personality, xix, xx, 16, 36, 50, 72, 85,
    88, 94-9, 123, 128, 135, 136,
    139, 141, 142, 143, 148, 154,
    164
    breakdown of, 123
    theories of, 96
petrification, 134, 154
phantasies, 75, 76, 88, 92, 94, 98, 141,
    144, 151, 157, 160
phenomena, see bodily, biological,
    cerebral, disease, individual,
    masochistic, mental, natural,
    physical, psychiatric, psychic,
    psychological, sadistic, social,
    symbolic, value-free social in-
    vestigation
phenomenological and existential prin-
    ciples in a medical framework,
    130-42

phenomenological approach, the,
    128-9, 155
Philosophy of As-If, 85
physical illness, 121, 132, 144, 161
physical phenomena, 68, 110, 161
physical reality, concepts and, 53-5
physicalism, 3, 10, 59, 109, 110
phobias, 13
Plague, The, 150
play therapy, 31
pleasure principle, the, 111
protoplasm, doctrine of, 10
psyche, the, xix, 62, 65, 66, 75-102,
    114, 128, 164 and passim
psychiatric diagnosis, framework of
    137-42
psychiatric knowledge, epidemiological,
    67-8
psychiatric social phenomena, 69
psychiatry
    community, 67, 70
    idea of social challenge in, 65-7
psychic determinism and freedom,
    94-9
psycho-analysis, xxi, 22, 78
psychobiology, social, 71-2
psychological medicine, theory in, 62-3
Psychologie der Weltanschauungen, 62
psychologism, 109
psychopath(s), 69, 70, 154
psychotherapeutic encounter, the
    154-60
psychotics, 32, 84, 151, 152, 153, 154,
    161
psycho-somatic conditions, 67, 74
psycho-somatic system, 49
public health education, 121
purposiveness, 12, 16, 19, 20, 21, 36,
    43, 56, 57, 59, 65, 97

rationalistic determinism, 126
reality, see: biological, empirical,
    organic, physical, psychic
refined carbohydrates, xxi, xxii, xxiii,
    26
reflexes, 11, 16
regulative function, 63
regulative judgement, 57, 58, 59
regulative principle, the, 62, 95
relatedness, 44
relationship, see: dialogical, doctor-
    patient, human, libidinal-object,
    monological, mother-baby,
    mother-child
religion(s), 90, 149, 163
resentment, xx, 69, 157, 161
response, 11, 16, 65, 93, 122, 126
responsibility, 128, 133, 136, 148, 160
reverie technique, 158

sadistic phenomena, 78

Sartre's ontologies, 146-8
satisfaction, 12, 97, 98
'Sciences of Psychiatry, The', 63
scientific theory, 46, 48, 49, 63
scientism, 120, 123, 128
schizoids, 30, 148
schizophrenia, 94, 132
schizophrenic, the, 30, 91, 94, 101, 139-41, 150, 154
security, 133, 134, 141, 154
self
    and 'not-self', 19
    archetypal, 89, 128, 143
    as agent, 130
    faith in, 149
    false, 146, 152
    healthy, true, 133
    integrity of, 142
    moral, 133, 143
    pseudo-, 125
    sick, demoralized, 133, 134
self-contempt, 136
self-destruction, 23, 135, 141, 147
self-love, 124
self-understanding, 55
selfhood, 150, 151, 152, 158
sensation, 53, 72, 94
sense-datum theory, 43
sexual aetiology of mental illness, 77
sexual development, 81
sexual excitement, 162
sexual instinct, 77, 78, 91, 124, 142, 143, 164
sexual love, 124
sexual perversions, 124
sexual trauma, 82
Sickness Unto Death, The, 155
Sisyphus, 150
situational treatment, 30, 31, 32
social actions, 66, 69-70
social challenge, 65-7, 70, 71, 72, 73, 75
    social conflict, 75
social environment, 67, 79
social evolution, 70-1, 84
social groups, 22, 23, 68
social habits, 71
social influences, 137
social life, deterministic-scientific approach to, 68-9
social mental health, 73
social milieu, 98, 137, 162
social mind, 66, 67, 73
social nexus, 136
social phantasy system, 136
social psychiatry, 31, 48, 64, 65-75, 84
social psychobiology, 71-2
social relations, 72, 73
social therapeutic clubs, 31, 32

society's attitude to mental patient, 69-70
solar penis and Greek papyrus, 91
soul, 62, 63
specific mechanistic-materialistic aproach, the, 49
specific mechanistic principle, the, 33
stimulus, 11, 12, 13, 16, 22, 24, 27, 30, 52, 59, 63, 78, 122, 123, 126, 137, 164
style of life, 84, 85, 86, 143
subconscious mind, 94
subconscious self, 29
subjective causality, 85
subjective ethical principle, 164
subjective experience, 75, 77, 81, 85, 129, 156
subjective striving, 144
subjective teleology, 86
substrate, *see*: biological, holistic principle, indifferent self-identical, 3, 10
suggestion
    holistic, 28-9
    laws of, 94, 95, 164
super-ego, 23, 78, 124, 125
superiority, 85, 86, 144, 145
symbol of individuation, 89
symbolic imagery, 88
symbolic phenomena, 91
symbolism, 76, 77-8, 81
synchronicity, 88
system(s), 5, 7, 48, 64, 65, 73, 74

teleological behaviour, 7
teleological concepts, 58, 90
teleological explanations, 4, 5, 17, 59, 97
teleological feature of life, 114
teleological judgement, 57, 58
teleological medico-ethical principle, 73
teleological metaphysics, 47
teleological principle, the, 18, 20, 24, 25, 26, 35, 36, 47, 48, 57, 60, 72, 75, 84
teleological metaphysics, 47
teleology, 16, 36, 57, 62, 64, 72-5, 83, 84, 86
telos, 17, 18, 47, 85
tension, 23, 73, 75
Textbook of Psychiatry, 138
theory, *see*: aggressive, libidinal, mental phenomena, metaphysical, personality, psychological, psychological medicine, scientific, sense-datum
therapeutic groups and clubs, 31, 32, 158, 159
totality, 63

transaction, behavioural definition of, 64
transcendental function of symbol, 89
transcendental objects, 44
transference, 160

unconscious, the, 69, 78, 82, 126, 128, 135, 142
unconscious, collective, 87, 88, 90, 91
unconscious conscience, 98
unconscious experience, 135, 142
unconscious fears, 70
unconscious feelings, 81
unconscious motives, 81, 82, 96
unconscious resentment, 69
'understanding psychology', 155, 156
universal essence, 3
universal harmony, 87
universals, xix, 109, 111
universe, ontological structure of, 43
'unlearning', 12
'Use and Abuse of Drugs', 33

value-free investigation of phenomena, 80
values, 71, 96, 119, 123, 125, 126, 129, 130, 133
vitalists, 24, 25
vitality, 35
vitamin deficiencies, xxiii
volition, 72

wholeness, xxii, 16, 26, 43, 44, 47, 48, 56, 64, 72, 89
whole person, the, xxi, 12
Wisdom of the Body, The, 19
withdrawn personalities, 30, 154
women in labour, hospital attitude to, 120-21

Yoga, 163